I Am Their Voice

I AM THEIR VOICE

A Guide for Caregivers and Advocates

JULIE MOORE

First Edition
Paperback ISBN: 978-1-955541-63-3
eBook ISBN: 978-1-955541-65-7
Hardcover ISBN: 978-1-955541-64-0
Library of Congress Control Number: 2025904567

Cover and Interior Design by Ann Aubitz

Published by FuzionPress
1250 E 115th Street
Burnsville, MN 55337
FuzionPress.com
612-781-2815

IN LOVING MEMORY

This book is dedicated to: Carol Prescott (1939–2023), Clint Prescott (1962–2023), as well as Ralph Prescott, Sr. (1933–2021)—three loving souls we will forever miss and long to see again when it is our time to leave this Earth.

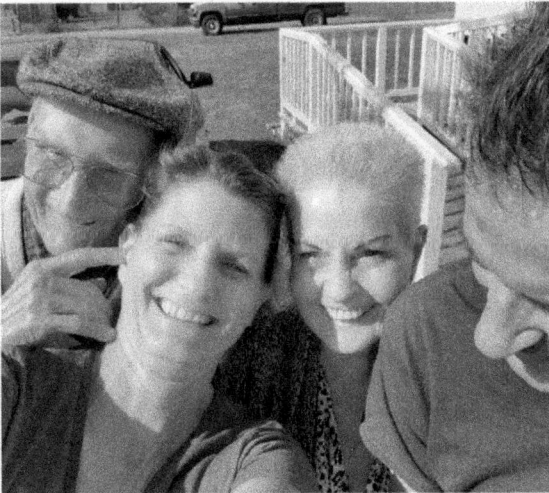

Ralph, Julie, Carol, Clint—2019

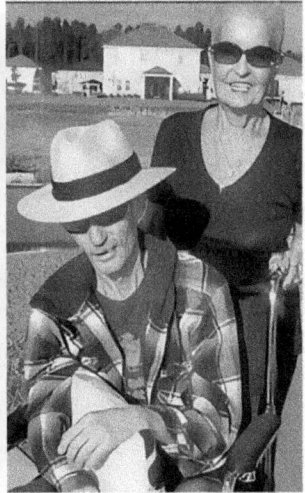

Carol and Clint—2021

ACKNOWLEDGEMENTS

I personally would like to thank those who were in my corner and whom I leaned on heavily as my support group throughout my time as a caregiver. Thank you for your prayers, words of encouragement, and for being my sounding board whenever I doubted my own strength and abilities. I am forever grateful for your support, kindness, and patience.

My love to you all.
My sisters and brother, Renée, Marcus, and Karla
Members of Grace and Faith Church, Tampa, Florida
My children, Kaitlyn and Adam
My husband, Charles
My closest friends, Hope, Mike, and Rachael
My military sisters, Holly, Theresa, Katherine, Angel, Camellia, Tracey, and Nannette

CONTENTS

FOREWORD

As a Board-Certified Elder Law Attorney[1] and a former caregiver to aging parents, I personally witness clients struggle with the daunting task of taking care of a loved one every day. Whether it is the sleep-deprived and anguished wife who is simply too exhausted, too sick, too emotionally spent caring for her husband with advanced Alzheimer's 24 hours a day, or the adult son who is busy taking care of his own kids in another state suddenly being thrust into making all the decisions and coordinating medical care and housing for his mother. As an only child, I too have been called upon to help my parents and know firsthand the emotional highs and lows that come with caregiving.

A little over two years ago, I met Julie Moore when she was throes of caring for her mother with stage four breast cancer and moving her into a local care facility. I was immediately impressed with her knowledge of her mother's needs and how to meet and pay for those needs, as well as her organization, and preparation for our meeting. My impressions were further confirmed when I helped her administer her mother's and brother's

---

[1] Board certified by the Florida Bar.

estates and affairs after their deaths. Throughout it all, she has been the model of composure and dignity with resourcefulness.

The book *I Am Their Voice* is the amazing story of her journey as caregiver to both her brother and her mother. It provides a very honest portrayal of the difficulties and blessings that come from being a caregiver. The book begins by defining dementia and describes how her loved one's reality began to change and how to navigate those changes. It also illustrates the challenges of dealing with medical personnel and facilities and the importance of advocacy. Furthermore, the book introduces public resources and government supports, as well as the once taboo subject as preparing for the end of life and what happens to family and belongings after death. Finally, the book ends with a poignant sighting of a beautiful red cardinal and dreams featuring her mother and her brother.

I Am Their Voice is a must-read for adults with aging or suddenly incapacitated or disabled loved ones – whether they be parents, grandparents, siblings, aunts, uncles, children, grandchildren, other relatives, friends, and neighbors. This book would also be very illuminating for the various professionals who service caregivers or patients, such as, attorneys, accountants, financial advisors, counselors, parish nurses, clergy personnel, care managers, nurses, home health aides, social workers, etc. Personally, this book made me laugh and cry. It was both educational and cathartic, resonating deeply with my own experiences as a caregiver.

I am profoundly grateful to Mrs. Moore for allowing me the opportunity to read this book when I did, following a period of caregiving for my father.

~Heidi M. Brown, Esq.

INTRODUCTION

Congratulations on taking a step in the direction of learning more about caring for your loved ones, or, if you are a medical professional, caring for someone in your charge! This book is about advocacy for another human being: learning to see the world through their eyes and making decisions that are in *their* best interests when they are no longer capable of doing so.

Caring for another human being comes at a great cost, and this book will not sugarcoat that price. It comes under the guise of finances, personal and mental health, personal expectations and livelihood, friendships, and family relationships.

The goal of this book is to share my experiences in these areas and provide possible and/or successful solutions. Everyone's situation is different. Therefore, not every response will fit yours, but it may put you on the right path and get you to your goal faster, so keep reading!

Through these experiences, I will share methods or actions I tried in my duties as a caregiver—some failed, some were successful. However, in many cases, it was the variety of training I have had and from which I drew knowledge that further helped me in those decisions.

I am a 30-year retired U.S. Army veteran, whose primary duty was in human resource management. The U.S. Army instilled in me the value of routines that helped me with time management, along with preparing myself mentally to manage stress. I learned how to research, find, interpret, and follow regulations. I learned the importance of processes and procedures, why I should save documents and ask questions that no one else may have thought important at the time, and how to stand up for myself and those around me. Additionally, when my children were little, I discovered that having routines, processes, and systems in place was beneficial for managing their time, their expectations, and my sanity!

When caring for adults with disabilities, this is no different. Establishing a schedule, as close to a routine as possible (this comes with exceptions), will provide a sense of stabilization for the disabled adult. Additionally, having a regular routine will give you, as the caregiver, a sense of control and an understanding of what's expected of you. Knowing how to research and find information will help you advocate for your loved one. Being a caregiver of not one, but two adults with disabilities put me in a variety of stressful situations. Caring for one loved one is tough enough, but if you find yourself in a position of caring for two people with special needs, you will need to be prepared—first mentally, then physically and emotionally—to not just manage but overcome that stress. I trust this book will help you with that.

I come from a family of six: one older sister (Renée), two older brothers (Clint and Marcus), a younger sister (Karla), and a brother (Corey). I will share a little about each of them, but the focus of this book will be on my oldest brother, Clint, and my mother, Carol.

In 2020, I moved both Mom and Clint in with me and became their full-time caregiver. Mom was still performing all of her, what I would soon come to learn as, "ADLs," or activities of daily living. This meant she was able to bathe herself, get herself dressed, take care of her toileting needs, and feed herself, whereas Clint could not. Mom had spent the previous ten years caring for her own mother with Alzheimer's, then herself with a breast cancer diagnosis, then her daughter-in-law, who also suffered from Alzheimer's, then Clint with early-onset dementia at age 54.

As I'm writing this, I am 56 years old and I often think about where Clint was at my age now, as he watched his world spin out of control. Clint was eventually given a more specific diagnosis of frontotemporal dementia. It is in fact the same diagnosis a very famous actor has been given, and his family has been living with, in just the last couple of years.

Between fighting her cancer, caring for both my sister-in-law and Clint, the stress of it all began showing on Mom. She was tired, 80 years old, a retired nurse, and needed someone to care for her. I was recently retired, and not only did it make sense for me to accept that responsibility, but I had also been seeking a new purpose in life and *needed* to step into this new role.

You may read this book and ask, "Are there cameras in my house, because you seem to know exactly what I'm going through!" No, but I really do know what you are going through, and I hope you find comfort and support in knowing that you are not alone. And if there is anything else you gain from reading this book, I hope it will be answers to the questions for which you have been seeking help for months, if not years. Another benefit may simply be having access to resources that no one has ever shared, in one common space. In that case, this book just became a valuable *must-read*!

If you need resources, keep reading; if you need ideas of possible solutions, keep reading; if you need to know that you are not losing your mind and you are not crazy, keep reading!

This is the first building block to your support group—and for more on that, keep reading!

PART ONE

PART ONE

WHAT IS EARLY-ONSET DEMENTIA?

We have all seen movies or read books where someone has dementia. Or maybe we have a friend with a family member who talks about their experience. But what is dementia? The Alzheimer's Organization gives a great depiction of what dementia is. It's like an umbrella with multiple **types** of dementia underneath. One of the most common types of dementia is Alzheimer's. Another type is frontotemporal dementia (FTD), a.k.a. frontotemporal lobar degeneration (FTLD) or Pick's disease. The additional research that has been done with FTD has shown it to be on a spectrum with subtypes. These subtypes include behavioral variant FTD, primary progressive aphasia, amyotrophic lateral sclerosis (ALS) and frontotemporal degeneration, corticobasal syndrome, and progressive supranuclear palsy. According to The Association for Frontotemporal Degeneration (AFTD), "they represent a group of brain disorders caused by degeneration of the frontal and/or temporal lobes of the brain" (https://www.theaftd.org/what-is-ftd/disease-overview). The diagnosis of "early-onset" dementia or Alzheimer's is given to anyone showing the signs and symptoms of either disease between the ages of 30 and 64.

Clint, a 24-year retired U.S. Air Force veteran, was diagnosed at age 54. He had been fired from his job, was unable to cook for himself, and could no longer manage his finances. His weight had significantly dropped, and he was struggling to complete sentences in a conversation. But no one really noticed his decline until he lost weight and began struggling with his speech. He was doing all he could to hide what he knew wasn't quite right with his mind and abilities, that he himself could not explain. It wasn't until he froze in the middle of the church stage, standing in a daze unaware of his brief pause, that his secret finally exposed. Speaking with a neighbor, the family began putting the puzzle pieces together; Clint was experiencing an urgent medical situation, if not an emergency, and they needed to get a doctor involved immediately.

After multiple MRIs, CTs, bloodwork, and a failed neurological-psychiatric examination, the family was initially told Clint was diagnosed with frontotemporal dementia (FTD)-primary progressive aphasia (PPA). "What the heck is that?!" we asked. We were given a few brochures on FTD and PPA and early-onset dementia, along with some homework for Clint to do to re-engage his faculties (e.g., drawing hands on a clock to represent a specific time, identifying pictures of fruits or animals, or filling in the blank of a sentence). The following was listed on his neuropsych exam as his full diagnosis:

- Frontal-temporal dementia-PPA
- Attention and concentration deficit
- Communication deficit
- Retrograde amnesia

- Anterograde amnesia
- Major depressive episode, severe, possibly psychotic

Needless to say, after all the tests, exams, and homework assignments, we were left with more questions than answers. The family was given a pamphlet and basically left to "figure this out on your own." None of this made sense! This was "Clint" for Christ's sake! The intelligent one! The good-looking one! The talented and outgoing one! This cannot be right! There must be another explanation. We questioned if he had a brain tumor, Lyme disease, "something" other than what we thought was an "old man's disease." Clint was only 54 years old!

The World Health Organization listed the following "Key Facts" on their website (https://www.who.int/news-room/fact-sheets/detail/dementia, March 15, 2023) regarding dementia cases worldwide:

Key facts:

- Currently more than 55 million people have dementia worldwide, over 60% of whom live in low- and middle-income countries. Every year, there are nearly 10 million new cases.
- Dementia results from a variety of diseases and injuries that affect the brain. Alzheimer disease is the most common form of dementia and may contribute to 60–70% of cases.
- Dementia is currently the seventh leading cause of death and one of the major causes of disability and dependency among older people globally.

- In 2019, dementia cost economies globally 1.3 trillion US dollars, approximately 50% of these costs are attributable to care provided by informal carers (e.g., family members and close friends), who provide on average five hours of care and supervision per day.
- Women are disproportionately affected by dementia, both directly and indirectly. Women experience higher disability-adjusted life years and mortality due to dementia but also provide 70% of care hours for people living with dementia.

Those statistics are truly alarming. The cost of care alone, just five years ago, was already over a trillion US dollars, with half of that cost being paid by family members and friends. Then, the fact that not only are women more likely to have dementia, but they provide 70% of the care hours for the family members living with it. Our family was included in those statistics.

We all aspire to be something when we grow up: a pro ball player, a lawyer, a doctor, a musician, or a teacher—usually a career that, for some reason, holds interest and fascination for us. Some of us have support systems and resources in place to help us become exactly who we want to be. However, many kids grow up without resources or mentors to set them on the path of success, limiting their choices of paths to follow. My siblings and I, in our own timing, found ourselves seeking a more structured environment than what we were growing up in and around.

My oldest brother, Clint, seemed to love life, and he embraced it the best he knew how. Like many adults, he had a lot of questions and doubts about life. He questioned whether he was making good or right decisions as an adult. He was trying to understand his religious path as well as navigate society at large.

Clint loved working with kids and teaching them to play soccer. He grew up playing soccer and drums in the marching band and was a talented artist. He liked listening to rhythm and blues and dancing, but he was also crazy smart. I remember him taking calculus in ninth grade. That was impressive to our family.

When I think of Clint, I remember him walking through the house with his drumsticks, drumming on the walls. Mom would yell at him to stop, but he would smile or giggle and keep on "tap-tap-tapping." In high school, he submitted one of his drawings to the local paper for a competition and he won! They posted his drawing in the next issue.

When he graduated high school, he joined the Air Force. The subject of higher education wasn't part of our family dialogue, we were very much a blue-collar family. I was 12 years old and vaguely remember him leaving for basic training. I don't remember it being a big deal, but I can never forget how exciting it was to know that his first duty station would be in Japan. Wow! To live in and experience another country!

We believe his symptoms of dementia began around 2014. The first to notice was someone who was very close to him, but she didn't know his family yet (not well enough to suggest a problem) and thought he just needed help managing some of his affairs, as any typical bachelor might. Some of the signs and symptoms of FTD, as shown on the AFTD website, include changes in behavior and personality that are not within their normal character. They may experience apathy and struggle with decision-making, speaking, or language comprehension. Outwardly, people with FTD appear normal, but neurodegeneration is happening inside their brain as it begins to rob the individual of who they once were. Clint's brain was shrinking. Can you imagine your brain shrinking? He was losing motor skills and other faculties, which increased his anxiety and grip on life as this disease lurked around inside.

Brain degeneration may be the cruelest of all diseases. You become trapped in your own mind, fighting—if not screaming to anyone who might possibly hear "you" on the inside—saying, "Wait! I'm here! —I'm here!"

CHAPTER ONE
UNDERSTANDING THEIR REALITY

When "Reality" Starts to Change

The day Clint walked into the recruiting office in Jacksonville, Florida, in 1980 and signed on the dotted line was the beginning of his 24-year career in the U.S. Air Force. After he enlisted, people came to our house asking questions about Clint, and they also talked to our neighbors. It was the background check for him to receive a top-secret clearance. That was a big deal in my 12-year-old eyes. We never knew what Clint's job in the military was. It was only recently, when I was looking through some of his military files, that I found a résumé on which he was working, where I finally learned he was a cryptologist—wow! A cryptologist deciphers secret code and can also encrypt information—how cool is that! He also learned Morse code and worked for the National Security Agency at Fort Meade, Maryland. I began wondering what sort of intelligence he deciphered. Oh, how I would love to ask him those questions now.

Clint served honorably in the military and served alongside other great service members, some of whom will share stories later in this book of good times with Clint. However, like many service members of that era, he neglected to seek medical care (mentally or physically) in fear of tarnishing his military record and losing his position, if not being forced out of the military. Clint loved the Air Force; he loved his job, and he was damn good at it! But he struggled with anxiety and elevated levels of stress. By not seeking the counseling needed to address these issues, he robbed himself of the benefits available only to veterans with a documented "service-connected" disability. I would later learn more about these benefits when Clint needed them most.

Clint did not remain in the cryptology job for long. I remember him telling me that "his first job in the military" (he wasn't allowed to divulge what he did) was a lot of stress, so he requested to retrain in medical administration. That landed him an assignment working in the Washington, DC, area, bouncing between the Pentagon, Andrews Air Force Base, and Bolling Air Force Base for most of his career. He then had an assignment in Biloxi, Mississippi, before finishing up his career, where he started it, in Japan. He retired in 2004 as a senior master sergeant.

In 2014, Clint reached out to me to help connect him to veteran resources while he was in between jobs and to help him with his résumé. I didn't know it at the time, but he had been fired from his job at the hospital, was living off his savings, and had withdrawn his retirement funds from his 401(k). I sent him as much information as I could, including reaching out to the local military base for assistance. I also shared it with Renée (our older sister), as she lived close to him (I was stationed in Kentucky) so that she could help too. I continued to try and help Clint as much as I could through email, and before I knew it, a year went by. By 2015, he still had no job and was beginning to decline mentally and physically. Renée noticed he was losing weight rapidly. But we had not yet connected these facts to Clint losing his job. Clint, on the other hand, was investing time in another job: the well-being of his inner self.

During 2015, Clint began attending Renée's church, and after about six months, she encouraged him to join the orchestra. He started playing drums for the church orchestra, where she already played the flute. Also, during this time, he entrusted her with his questions about God and learning to hear from God. She explained the importance of prayer and "listening" for God's answers in the way of feeling a stir in your spirit or hearing a small, still voice. Shortly after, an opportunity for such an exercise presented itself. Clint had been driving an old pickup truck, and he needed a new car before the truck gave out on him. He had saved his money and was ready to buy. He began praying about getting a new vehicle—where to buy it and when to buy it. He listened. He was driving home one day and saw the car "he" wanted, but then he heard it: "Not now." No, not an audible voice, but something in his spirit—a whisper telling him, "No, that's not it." So, Clint waited. Then, when he was leaving church on another day, he heard, "That one. Go to that dealership." He looked up and sure enough, there was a car dealership across from the church. So, he went and found the car he had always wanted: a Cadillac.

For those of you who may be questioning, "Why would God tell you which dealership to go to, much less speak to you about buying a car?" the answer is that God works in mysterious ways and in his time. Turns out the salesman also attended the church Clint and Renée went to. They never saw the man at church and had never met him before that day. But in attending the same church, God gave Clint favor with the salesman, and he offered Clint a better deal. On top of that, once the salesman learned Clint was retired military, God showed him favor again and the salesman reduced the price even more.

The point is, Clint grew in his faith.

Clint was amazed at his developing relationship with God, which was a blessing because of the year he had experienced. And it was one more bond our family shared. First, Marcus (my second oldest brother) turned over a new leaf when he was younger and became a teacher of the Bible. He had insights and understanding of scripture that would blow our minds. Then Renée had her own testimony and had, on many occasions, heard the voice of the Lord and had a very strong relationship with God. As for me, I very much believed in God and heard stories of people having those types of experiences and relationships with God but never personally experienced it. I believed it could happen; it just hadn't happened to me yet. My life was very busy, and our family was in and out of church. I often worked on the weekend—50 to 60 hours a week—so my relationship with God was scarce, at best. I still believed in God, and I knew he was still "there"; I just didn't have time to talk to him. But Clint became witness to the power of the Holy Spirit and leaned into that power.

One night in 2016, Renée called me with concern about something she observed with Clint at church. They had just finished practicing, and Renée and Clint were putting away the music stands and books. Renée left Clint on the stage to gather up the stands while she took the books back to the band room. After about 10 minutes, when Clint never came in with the stands, Renée went back out to the sanctuary and found him standing in the middle of the stage in a trance of some sort, just standing in one spot, frozen.

Renée called his name and asked what he was doing. He responded with, "Uh, I don't know. Am I supposed to be doing something?" She also shared that over the previous few weeks, she had noticed he had lost a lot of weight and didn't think he was eating. Renée then had Clint over for a cookout and noticed he was struggling to find words to finish a sentence. She asked me to call and talk to him to get my opinion. I immediately called Clint to have a casual "Hey, how's it going?" conversation. Sure enough, he was struggling to finish a sentence. Red flag.

My first thought was that maybe he had had a stroke. I sent Renée some information on a "home test" she could do to check if he had had a stroke but told her that she needed to go to his house to perform the exercises. She had a full-time job, and Clint lived across the river from her. It was about four days after our phone call before she could get over to him. She called me that Saturday and said he passed each exercise except for the speech.

Although relieved he had not had a stroke, there was still something going on, and he needed to go to a doctor immediately. While at Clint's, Renée noticed he had no food in his kitchen except for Little Debbie snack cakes and Cokes. She asked Clint when the last time was that he ate a good meal, and he didn't know; he couldn't answer the question of *time* —another red flag.

He said his neighbor Kathy would invite him to dinner sometimes. We also found out he was behind on his bills, and Renée learned that Kathy had been helping him pay his bills too, both by balancing his checkbook, mailing the payment out, and on occasion giving him money to pay his bills. So, Renée took him to the grocery store to buy groceries.

While there, he wanted to buy himself a Coke, but instead of handing the cashier the $20 bill in his wallet, he used his debit card. When Renée suggested he just pay with the cash, he later told her that he was afraid the cashier would cheat him out of his money and not give the correct change back (paranoia—another red flag). Clint confided later that he couldn't do the math to determine if the correct cash was returned, so he just used his debit card (inability to do a simple math calculation). Several red flags immediately went up, all at once, because, as I mentioned earlier, Clint had a brilliant mind! Math was never an issue. For him to lose confidence in mentally calculating the cost of a soda from $20 was unheard of!

When Renée shared that with me, I asked her if he had gone to the doctor yet, and she said that he never scheduled the appointment. I then urged her to make the appointment for him and be prepared to take him to the appointment to ensure he went. A CT scan was ordered, and the initial prognosis was that a cyst was sitting at the base of his spine and fluid was building. Clint had been making comments that he didn't socialize anymore and believed he was just losing a perishable skill of talking and carrying on a conversation. He was trying to justify why he was struggling to complete a sentence or recall words. Over and over, he would blame the old boss who had fired him from his job in 2014. Clint talked about the level of stress he was under and that the boss would always yell at him. We believe that Clint was in the beginning stages of FTD and was struggling to do his job. From the boss's point of view, Clint was becoming incompetent, so he fired Clint. Clint really didn't understand what was happening to him, to his mind, and was reaching for some explanation—just something to give it all meaning, anything to explain this decline. Once again, our siblings rallied together to set up a phone schedule for people to call him on a regular basis to help get him back in the habit of talking and having conversations with people until the doctors figured out what to do next.

After the CT scan, Clint's doctor ordered an MRI, which showed nothing wrong. But when a neurologist repeated the MRI, this one showed his brain had shrunk. The doctors then got him in for a neurological-psychiatric examination. The exam should have taken approximately two hours, but after six hours of Clint struggling to complete the tasks given, the examiner ended the exam.

It was then, mid-2016, two years after symptoms began, that our brother Clint, now age 54, was officially diagnosed with early-onset frontal-temporal dementia (FTD). We were in denial. Clint had also tested positive for Lyme disease, so the doctor gave him one round of antibiotics, re-tested him, and got a negative result. I still question if it was Lyme all along and not dementia. The two MRIs that were taken appeared to be in conflict, and Clint had two 120-pound German shepherds that would sometimes sleep in his bed—maybe they brought in a tick. I just did not want to believe my brother had dementia, especially at such a young age.

Learning that Clint was being diagnosed with early-onset FTD was a hard pill to swallow. Talk about having your world come to a sudden stop! Our family was in denial and could not believe what we were being told. My heart ached for my brother. I wanted so badly to prove the doctors wrong; our whole family wanted to. From that day forward, our lives will never be the same.

The year 2016 proved to be an incredibly challenging, stressful year for my family. Soon after the doctors diagnosed Clint with Lyme disease, my own son went hiking and picked up a tick. Within a week, he began presenting neurological decline. When he finally found the tick and told my husband what he was experiencing, my husband took him to the doctor, where he was diagnosed with Lyme disease and placed on antibiotics.

I was a student in a required, high-stress, intense military course at the time and trying to manage phone calls about Clint when I learned about my son. I had stepped outside of class to take a call from my son's doctor, and that's how I found out he had Lyme disease. My husband didn't tell me what was going on, to not add to my stress, but the doctor's office didn't know that. I was standing in the bathroom at the academy, and I just slid down the wall onto the floor and began weeping from everything that was going on. And, as if that wasn't enough, about a month later, my mother learned the cancer had returned to her spine and she was diagnosed with stage 4 cancer. Adding insult to injury, her trailer burned down. She moved in with Marcus, which turned out to be helpful for him too, as Janice, his wife, could no longer be left home alone, as she herself had Alzheimer's. Mom, the forever caregiver, continued to care for Janice and undergo her own chemo and radiation therapy.

In 2017, a family decision was made to move Clint to Georgia with Marcus and Mom. I hear what you are thinking: "Why put so much on your mom?" The guilt within me continues from that decision. But we found ourselves stuck between a rock and a hard place. We weren't a family of means. Renée had a full-time job that came with the health insurance needed for her and her husband. I was on active duty with the military. I did apply for what's known as a "compassionate" reassignment, requesting to be transferred to an assignment in Jacksonville to be closer to Clint and care for him myself. However, the Army saw that I had other siblings and made the decision to deny the request. Karla (my younger sister) was married to an active-duty sailor, living in another state and physically she would not have been able to manage Clint, who was 5 feet 10 inches, where she was only 5 feet 2 inches. Our youngest brother, Corey, was neither available nor dependable. Trust me, when I said it was a family decision, we discussed all the options, everyone's availability and capabilities, and moving Clint to live with Mom and Marcus was the most viable option.

We already had Clint's driver's license revoked because he had lost his peripheral vision and he was no longer safe to drive, much less live alone. Mom eventually bought a new trailer that she and Clint moved into. Mom, at the age of 77, was surely covered with God's grace as she endured the return of cancer—and the treatments for it, continued to care for her daughter-in-law and now her oldest son.

My life in the Army was keeping me on my toes. I was stationed at Fort Knox in 2010 and had three different assignments from 2010 to 2017 while there. My last assignment was at an Army Reserve Training Academy, where I served as a chief instructor. I had just been transferred to that role when we received Clint's official diagnosis —I was torn between my contractual obligations to the Army and the love for my family. The best I could do, the most I could give, was take a week of leave (vacation time) to go stay with Clint, observe him in his environment, and relay those observations to his neurologist. I did that on two separate occasions in 2016. This was how we knew about his loss of peripheral vision, eating habits, and repetitive or odd behaviors. Then my younger sister, Karla, did the same thing. She took a week to stay with him, cook, and clean for him and observe. Renée began driving 30 minutes to his house to pick him up and take him to his doctor's appointment. One of my aunts who lived in the area also took him to a couple of his appointments. It was truly a village-like effort to get to the bottom of whatever was happening to Clint.

During my two stays observing Clint in 2016, I would get up when he got up, and I would stay in the background, watching his routine. I entered "Clint's" world, and this is what it looked like:

- At 5:30 a.m., he would wake up and pour two cups of coffee. His neighbor and girlfriend, Kathy, lived just two doors down from him. He committed to having coffee with her every morning before she left for work. He loved Kathy, trusted her, and wanted to make sure she knew and felt his love and gratitude for her and all she had done for him, especially when he began to decline. Kathy has two boys, and I knew Clint tried to be a positive male figure in their lives. But it wasn't until recently that I learned of Clint's devotion to those boys and their love and gratitude toward Clint. There was a reciprocal relationship of trust and gratitude between Clint, Kathy, and her boys.
- 6:00 a.m.: Clint had two full-blooded German shepherds. They weighed 120 lbs. each. After having coffee with Kathy, Clint would walk the dogs. But getting them ready to walk was interesting to watch. First, imagine the size of the dogs, whose names were Garren and Tanzer. Now imagine their eagerness to go potty! Clint kept their leashes hanging in the coat closet by the front door. One was retractable (why a retractable leash for a 120 lb. dog?! I don't know), and the other was a regular leash. He would give them the command to sit so he could put the leash on. They would sit behind him, and Clint would get one hooked up, then

turn around to hook the other up. The problem was that he would sort of bump into the dog he needed to leash, causing it to stand and move out of the way. So, when Clint turned, he could no longer "see" where the dog was, and he kept turning in circles, getting frustrated. I finally spoke up and asked, "Clint, what are you trying to do?" Of course, I already knew from observation what he wanted to do, but I needed to hear him articulate it. Clint said, "I'm trying to get their leash on, but they keep moving and I can't see where they are!" At first, I told Clint that Garren was right next to his foot and asked if he could see him. Clint was frustrated and said, "No, he keeps moving," so I offered to help. After that, they finally left, following about 20 minutes of turning in circles.

- 6:45-7:00 a.m.: Clint prepared the dogs' food. First, he located their bowls and placed them on the stove —a glass-top black stove. He then pulled out a can of cat food and set it on the counter next to the stove. Clint then began searching for something. He opened and closed the pantry numerous times, then the fridge, then looked around the kitchen floor and hallway. Finally, after about five minutes of this, I asked, "Clint, whatcha doing?" Very flustered by this point, he said, "I can't find their bowls!" Confused, I asked, "The cat bowl?" To which he incredulously said, "No! The dog bowls. I already fed the cat!" So, without pointing, I told him they were on the stove, but he could not see the bowls. The black, glass top acted as an invisible shield. He stared intently, so I asked, "See them?" He said, still frustrated and with an incredulous "Noooo, I don't!" I took his hand and placed it on the bowls. I then suggested he use the granite counter and help move them there. "There, is that better? Can you see the bowls better here?" He said he could and continued with feeding the dogs.

While we were trying to figure out what was going on with Clint, I started researching everything I could about Alzheimer's, Lyme, and other neurological diseases. In one of my findings, I learned that some dementia patients' vision is affected in such a way that they cannot see items when sitting on certain colors. The Alzheimer's Organization states, "Changes in visual and spatial abilities may make it tough for someone with dementia to distinguish food from the plate or the plate from the table. It can help to use white plates or bowls with a contrasting color place mat." This applies not just to food. It is the color on which the item is sitting, and I tested this theory with Clint with the dog bowls on the black top stove. This disease just continued to amaze me and discourage me at the same time. I wanted to just make it all stop, but I couldn't. So, the next best thing was to learn about it, understand it, and learn how to make Clint's new world as comfortable as possible.

Once Clint's official diagnosis came in, before we made the decision to move Clint in with Mom and after my stay with him, Renée and I met with his neighbor Kathy to fill her in on everything we had learned from the doctors and our observations of Clint. We knew Kathy was more than just his neighbor; he had told us so. Clint loved Kathy very much. He cried knowing what was going on with him and saw the love of his life slipping away. For as long as he lived in his home, he continued to make her coffee every morning and would take walks with her, and she would make him dinner. They would go to church together and sometimes go to her parents for cookouts or to watch football games. Nonetheless, Clint was in a precarious position, and we needed to find out exactly where they were in their relationship.

It was the first time I had met Kathy. My first impressions were that she was a very sweet person who was very concerned about Clint's welfare and very much in love with him. She believed he was her soul mate and talked of how big of a role he played in her two boys' lives. She had two teenage boys and a full-time job as a professor at a local college. I have been told I can come across as overbearing, but it's a perception based on my preference to be direct to save time. My sister Renée is the opposite, so she was with me to keep me balanced. Renée is very much a comforter regardless of the situation. I can be a comforter—just to be clear. However, I considered the urgency of the matter and chose to get down to brass tacks sooner than later. The subject at hand was not a topic to tiptoe around.

Clint had a life-changing condition that would require *a lot* of medical care, and *a lot* of demand placed on whomever took the role as caregiver. I needed to know if Kathy was prepared to take on that role, or if practically she could. I wasn't ugly about it, not at all! This was our brother, and *his* welfare was our utmost concern. We needed to know if Kathy was ready and willing to do all that was required to see it through. And if she was not, to assure her, "That's okay." Becoming a full-time caregiver is a *huge* "ask" of anyone and not to be taken lightly.

Kathy had two teenage boys, a full-time job, and her whole life ahead of her. Although Clint was prepared to be with her till, he died, we also believed he would want her to give her attention to those two boys. Clint loved those boys as if they were his own. We knew that. It was a choice—a very hard choice—and we wanted to give her permission to make a very hard choice without any regret or blowback from the family. We wanted her to know she didn't hold the full responsibility of caring for Clint. We believed it was our responsibility to ensure he was taken care of but included her in the decision. Kathy cried; we all cried. This was tough!

Kathy decided to give her full attention to her two boys but continued to assist with getting Clint to appointments and picking up prescriptions for him. She continued to have coffee with him and cook for him, tidying up his place as needed and doing laundry, helping with the homework he got from the doctors. They would still take walks, holding hands, looking into each other's eyes, and saying "I love you"—until we had to move him to live with Mom. Clint had a cell phone and would text Kathy every day. It wasn't long before those messages were nothing more than gibberish, as Clint began losing fine motor skills.

Choosing to Be a Full-Time Caregiver

I'm not sure if anyone "decides" to be a caregiver growing up. At face value, the day-to-day tasks don't exactly look to be all that appealing if you were looking at a brochure in your high school counselor's office. The job description is extensive; the requirements are very demanding for your time. Your physical and emotional strength, not to mention your mental acuity, will be challenged daily. It is truly a choice—and it was Mom's choice when she agreed to take care of her oldest son, even though she was 77 years old. Regardless, she cared for her own mother and her daughter-in-law and managed her own health, battling breast cancer. And it was my choice, without question, when the time came for Mom to pass the baton to someone else, whether she knew she needed to or not. Whatever your reasons for assuming the role of caregiver for your loved one, know that they are fully aware of the sacrifice you are making and the challenges you have accepted as your new reality. Just know that all you have been through in your life, up to this point, has most certainly prepared you for it. You need only to reflect on your life to realize that everything happens for a reason. We may not know that reason now, but it will soon be revealed, and you are right where you're supposed to be.

Here is my reflection.

Leaning into military service seemed natural to our family. Our dad, an uncle, a cousin, both my older brothers, and I served in the military, and even my oldest sister followed a military-structured program. Daddy served in the Navy during the Korean War; he served for about six years. My brother Marcus, the "number three child," joined the Navy as a welder. The trade skills served him well when he got out and helped him as a Walmart distribution center maintenance manager.

Our oldest sister, Renée, was given the opportunity to join the Junior Reserve Officer Training Corps (JROTC) in high school. Although the reason for joining JROTC was to transfer to a school outside of our district, she had to choose to either take a foreign language not offered in our district or join an organization that offered structure and discipline—two characteristics she was already familiar with as a competitive baton twirler and disciplined flutist. Renée understood the importance of self-discipline, focus, and structure. JROTC's mission is to teach students citizenship, leadership, character, and community service. Those teachings gave Renée the foundation and training to set her on the path of owning one of the most well-known and successful baton-twirling schools in the nation and gave her the skills she still uses today in her current career as a senior representative of a nationwide pool company.

Music was another "discipline" our family appreciated, beginning with our father. He set the stage for the love of music in our family. Daddy played guitar, sang in a country band, and would play gigs in bars from Florida to Alabama. His day jobs included random ones, everything from working in a grease factory to working at a dry cleaner's. Once he joined a local church, got saved, and was baptized, he traded in the bar scene and began playing for the Lord, writing, singing, and even recording his Southern gospel music. Renée played the flute all through school. She learned how to play the piccolo and was selected to play in the all-county band in high school. She continued her love of music, playing for multiple churches throughout Jacksonville in her adult life. Daddy wrote her a song for one of her baton routines when she was just getting started, and just before he passed away, she played it for him on her flute. Clint played drums in school and quads in marching band. He also played a couple of gigs with our dad and played for his and Renée's church shortly before his diagnosis. I played the bassoon for one year and switched to playing flute for two years in junior high school. Marcus never played an instrument, unless you call a Chevy block engine his instrument of choice—he loved to tinker with his hands. And let's not forget dancing! We all loved to dance! Clint especially loved disco music and all the pop songs. We loved going to dance clubs, where we would just dance the night away! Music: it was in our bones. Disco, classical, hip-hop, classic rock, country, bluegrass—we loved it all. Music would come to prove to be the passageway that would allow Clint to hold on to reality a little bit longer.

Mom was always the caregiver. She served as a waitress for many years before attending a community college to become a licensed practical nurse (LPN). She was a single parent by then. She worked in nursing homes and hospitals, then eventually settled on and retired as a private duty nurse, where she worked for patients who were paraplegic or quadriplegic in their homes. I will share more about Mom's story a little later, but I can see how her example planted a seed within each of us.

I have shared my reflections on our upbringing and my relationship with Clint. But I realize that may not be enough for you and me to truly relate regarding managing life's challenges while serving as a caregiver. So, please allow me to pause for a moment and share a little more about me and grant you a peek into my own personal challenges—before, during, and after serving as a full-time caregiver to Clint and our mom.

I'll do my best not to bore you with every minute detail of my life. So, I will focus on and highlight specific points and/or specific people I believe have shaped me into the person I am today, not to mention giving me the training I needed to be Clint and Mom's caregivers. I have always said, "We are who we are, and we are where we are, because of the choices and decisions we have made, and the people in our life we allow to influence those choices and decisions." I remind myself of this during times of success or what appears to be failure or a setback. It allows me to retrace my steps and analyze what went right or wrong.

Leaning on Our Past to Push Forward

I may not have a PhD, but I love those who do because they are the ones who do the research and studies to generate theories to understand how or why things work. Their minds are always curious and seek the unknown, teaching us a new or different perspective of the functionality of a scientific principle or a process or system. I find myself enthralled with books on different studies of psychology, leadership, communication, or the mind. They open my mind to new possibilities of how to be a better human being, care for our body and our mind, especially how certain medications and foods affect our bodies. These books have opened my mind and perspective to many things we face in life and, I believe, have helped me make better choices and decisions, especially as a caregiver. I'd like to believe I'm a little smarter from reading them.

There are a few studies that discuss the importance of a child's first seven or eight years of life on their brain development and how that sets the stage for their maturing later in life, if not the type of person they will become. I mention this because I remember loving to write poetry (if we can call it that) or create my own cards to give to "friends" for their birthday. I could remember all my friends' and family's birthdays. This was my way of being a friend or asking someone to be my friend. But, as we know, sometimes kids can be cruel. Sometimes my cards were received and appreciated, but most times they were criticized and misunderstood, so I got a lot of laughs or jabs at how weird I was. If you've never read the book *Tribe* by Sebastian Junger, it is a great read. The author points out:

"We have a strong instinct to belong to small groups defined by clear purpose and understanding – tribes. This tribal connection has been largely lost in modern society but regaining it may be the key to our psychological survival."

Even children search for a tribe, a place to belong. That is what I believe I was doing — trying to find my place in the world, even at 7 and 8 years old. By third grade (7 years old), I discovered softball and began filling my spare time with softball and cheerleading (depending on the season) or baton twirling, which was year-round. I was involved in all three sports until my senior year of high school. It was within these sports that I found my tribes, places where I fit in. Each organized sport taught me teamwork, discipline, fitness, a sense of accomplishment, and friendships. Where else could I possibly find these elements in my adult life, except in the military? I didn't join immediately after high school. I needed to taste the freedom of adulting until I found myself needing three "hots and a cot" (three meals a day and a place to lay my head)! I joined the military at age 20.

When I joined the U.S. Army, I met my first husband at my first duty assignment. We had chemistry between us and thought we were ready to move in together. Unfortunately, we both were living in barracks on base and barely at the rank of specialist (E-4), which meant we would need permission to move off base — permission we both knew would not be given unless we were married. And getting married is exactly what we did! We grabbed two of our friends, went to the justice of the peace, to serve as witnesses, and "Ta-da!" got married. Although not the best reason to get married, we did give the marriage effort. However, being in our 20s, we were still discovering who we were — the research that our brains don't fully mature till 25 wasn't out (or I hadn't read about it yet). We were still trying to grow up ourselves on top of learning to care for another human being and willing to put their concerns ahead of our own. The marriage ended just shy of ten years, but the joy that came out of that marriage was a beautiful little girl named Kate.

When I met my second husband (also military), it was as if the waters had parted, the skies had cleared, and the angels descended on our presence (can you hear the heavenly choir singing yet?). We knew in our hearts that we each had found our soulmate. Charles and I had a connection that neither of us could truly explain, and that connection only grew stronger over the next 20 years. Charles was not just another military man in my life. He was a man with a focus and determination to achieve anything he set out to achieve. Next to his handsome face, deep brown eyes, and charming smile, he was a man with goals who acted toward those goals, which made him even more attractive and sexy in my eyes.

We met in Wisconsin, and within eight months of dating, found ourselves in front of the justice of the peace saying, "I do." Yes! Again. Second marriage, but no wedding (money saved!). We soon had our first child together, a son we named Adam, after the first man of the Bible. Charles was the doting father, giving thanks to God, praying blessings over Adam, and committing his soul back to God immediately after he was born. Charles was so proud to be a dad. Those are just the highlights of how our journey began. Know that we have faced all the typical challenges that young couples face with kids, both with and sometimes without grace.

Charles joined the military at age 17 and found his tribe. As an intelligent and driven man, he is not one to accept "no" for an answer for something he wants or believes he can achieve or feels he, or even someone else, deserves. He served with the 82nd Airborne (his "tribe") during Desert Shield-Desert Storm operations in the Gulf War. After being medically retired from the military, he did whatever needed to be done to continue to provide for our family. Added to his résumé are real estate investor, drone pilot, corporate trainer and training developer, project manager, and scrum master. At the time of writing this book, he started his own screen business, replacing lanai and pool cage screens. Within two months, it replaced the income he was making at his previous corporate job! Maybe "driven" is an understatement for a man who just won't stop at the word "No."

During my first ten years of military service, I served as a dental assistant. I enjoyed what I did, but over time, I found myself in somewhat of a rut. It became too routine, and I didn't feel as though I was growing professionally. I love telling people "I got tired of sucking spit and cleaning up after the doctor!" LOL! That's pretty much what a dental assistant (at least back then in the military) did. I could've applied for more advanced training to be a dental hygienist, but I knew I wanted to challenge my brain more. Learning more about teeth and gums and plaque no longer interested me. I retrained into the field of human resources. As nerdy as it sounds, researching regulations, studying, and writing policies, learning to deep-dive into a situation under investigation, problem solving, identifying a root cause, or learning and establishing systems and processes or procedures was right up my alley! The last twenty years of my military career were served as a human resources (HR) specialist/supervisor. When Charles and I met, I had just switched over to HR. A couple of years after we married, we both were assigned to Fort Jackson, SC. I had been released from active duty to give birth to our son, so I was serving as a reservist, and we were assigned to the same unit.

The chemistry that Charles and I had apparently showed up in unprovoked ways, as one of our fellow soldiers hilariously pointed out to us during a training event. The commander was conducting a briefing that required Charles, the operations NCO (noncommissioned officer), to discuss the upcoming training classes the soldiers needed to complete. Then I, the HR NCO, was reviewing the soldiers' requirements to update their annual physical exam and their military records review, to prepare for upcoming promotion boards. At one point in the briefing, both Charles and I were in tandem when we began tag-teaming almost in rapid fire, naming off the policies and regulations that governed all these requirements. After that briefing, a senior enlisted officer, the first sergeant in the organization, came up to Charles and me (privately) and asked in a low voice for only us to hear, "Do y'all recite regulations as foreplay, because that was romantic as hell?" We burst out laughing and were rolling in tears! The first sergeant just nonchalantly walked away after saying it! Oh, my goodness, we have gotten a laugh out of that ever since! But that was us!

I had the honor of serving as an assistant inspector general at an Engineering Command. I loved it! If you don't know what an Inspector General (IG) is or does, they are an entity that serves the greater good, ensuring regulations and policies are being enforced and not violated. This can be achieved through regular inspections, ensuring staff are following all requirements in a policy or regulation, receiving a whistleblower complaint of fraud or other serious violation, and investigating the charges. The line crosses over to the attorneys when the complaint becomes criminal, so we often worked alongside attorneys.

Working in IG, I learned how to investigate a complaint (which included writing a lot of reports), how to conduct an inspection (to ensure policies and regulations were being followed), and taught leaders how to conduct an inspection of their subordinate commands, ensuring policies, guidelines, and timelines were being met. I also learned how to better control my emotions by listening to the details of a complaint and understanding there is always two sides to every story—okay, three sides: the person making the complaint, the person on the other side of that complaint, and then the truth somewhere in between. It also opened my eyes and ears more, and I learned to read between the lines of what was being said or hear the undertones of desperation and despair. I understood the importance of a compassionate leader who knows their soldiers. Little did I know how my experience as an IG would come into play serving as a caregiver. The research skills, coupled with curiosity to ask hard questions, helped me when communicating with medical personnel.

I then had an opportunity to work directly with general officers, or "generals." Imagine working with Fortune 100 company CEOs directly—better yet, make that the chairman (the chairman can fire the CEO). For some folks, this would be a cause for panic at this point: working with a high-level official, and I was no different. I was an enlisted soldier at the rank of sergeant first class, with an assignment working with officers at the rank of colonel to major general, and their enlisted counterparts were command sergeants major, the highest enlisted rank in the military. I was confident in my job and the skills I would be bringing to the table. Especially coming off the IG assignment, my confidence was boosted. So, instead of walking into this new role afraid of what the generals would think or say or do to me, I reminded myself of what my skills were, and, at the end of the day, *they* "needed" my skillset.

My job was to advise them on regulation and policy; their job was to decide on what to do with that information. I became the senior personnel leader for the General Officer Selection Board and served there for four years. I completed my Master of Science degree in Performance Improvement and earned two certifications: a green belt and black belt in Lean Six Sigma. I developed great relationships and rapport with many of those general officers, who came to appreciate and respect my work, receiving multiple awards from each of their commands. If that doesn't make you walk a little taller—well, I certainly did!

This role prepared me with the understanding that although someone has had more training than me (i.e., doctors), they hold only a piece of the puzzle. When it came to my brother, or even my mother, I held all the other pieces, and the doctors needed me to fill in the gaps. Doctors give a prognosis based on the evidence in front of them: a mere snapshot in time and what previous studies and/or their experiences have shown. As a caregiver, I provided them with what they didn't know or couldn't see to help them prescribe the best solutions for my loved ones.

Another one of my favorite assignments was serving as chief instructor of a course teaching every human resource person in the U.S. Army Reserve. That could be an enlisted soldier, an officer, or a civilian (nonmilitary personnel) who worked in an HR capacity within the U.S. Army Reserve. This assignment was challenging for me because I had just worked four years with the General Officer board, which meant I lost four years of whatever had been going on in the field of human resources.

The field of human resources changed databases twice during those four years, so I did not have any training in them. But I was in charge. I, myself, had received a promotion to master sergeant. To say I doubted myself was an understatement. Not only did I have to teach topics I had never used, but I also had to lead my instructors, prepare the course schedule, and manage a team that was falling apart long before I arrived. I quickly had to prioritize my efforts, and that began with learning about my team and their needs, then jumping on just as quickly to the lessons I needed to get spun up on. There were many challenges with that assignment, and I learned some hard lessons, as any leadership position will teach you. Nonetheless, I was able to walk away with the respect of not only my peers but my superiors as well.

The takeaway from this assignment that I was able to use as a caregiver was listening, reviewing all the information in front of me, and then acting. I realized that listening to each doctor and specialist who treated my brother or mother was paramount in them receiving the best care "for them." Listening was crucial because, often, each doctor or specialist would not consider everything that was going on with the patient sitting in front of them. I found myself having to educate doctors (yes, really) on alternative theories of what may or may not be happening with either Clint or Mom at a given time. Doctors see many, many patients a day. They are not feasibly able to understand all that may be going on with a patient or changes that have happened since their previous visit. If we allow the doctor to make a judgment call, solely on face value of what they may be witnessing in the moment, it could be detrimental to your loved one. **You are their**

voice. You must be able to speak for your loved ones when they can't.

My last and final assignment before I retired was serving as the administrative assistant to the Command General and Command Sergeant Major of the Army Reserve Medical Command. I was the type of person who would take the bull by the horns, hitting the ground running. I took my role seriously and sought out ways to improve systems and processes while serving as the gatekeeper to my Command Sergeant Major. I would soon learn my value to the soldiers in the organization and the respect they had for my knowledge and awareness of regulations and policies. Both my peers and leaders from other departments in the organization trusted my input and, in some circles, gave me a seat at the table. If you've never read Leaders Eat Last by Simon Sinek or Lean In by Sheryl Sandberg, they are a must-read! Both were my guides to reaching the achievements I did reach during my 30-year military career. And they continued to serve me as a caregiver. These books taught me that my voice mattered and offering a different perspective on an issue can often be the right solution for everyone in the room.

Every time I went to a doctor's appointment with Clint or my mom, I made sure I always had a seat at the table. Honestly, there are many doctors (I call "good" doctors) who wish their patients would take that seat. Doctors don't always have the right answer, if an answer at all. They've taken all the classes, read all the studies, but every individual is just that—an individual. Therefore, what may work for one patient may not work for another.

So, speak up! Don't be afraid to say what you are thinking.

Ask questions!

There is no such thing as a "stupid question" when you are seeking to understand something about a disease or what is going to be in the best interest of the person for whom you are caring. If it's a new medication, ask, "What are the side effects?" and discuss if those side effects will help or harm: improve a situation or create a whole other issue to deal with?

Going back to my marriage to Charles, we weren't perfect nor was our marriage perfect, although many of our friends and family may have sometimes put us on a pedestal. Truth is, there is no perfect marriage or family. Every family has drama; regardless of the circumstances, there are just different circumstances to navigate. But it is how we choose to face those challenges and how we communicate that determines our future, only to face the next path of challenges another day. I thought, just as my family thought, Charles and I communicated well, better than most. We are both educated and well-read when it comes to the topic of communication.

Yet, somewhere along the way we stopped communicating and sharing. After a little over 19 years of marriage, a whole new path presented itself. A path that, although it may have surfaced in the far corners of our minds at one point or another, became a reality and we had to deal with it. I had to deal with it. As we began making plans for our 20-year anniversary, preparing for my upcoming retirement and a move to Florida, Charles decided that he wanted a divorce. That divorce was final near the end of 2018, and I retired from the Army in 2019. To say my world was turned upside down is just the tip of the iceberg.

We had bought an RV in preparation for our retirement, so I decided to move into that RV and lived there for over two years. Charles has his own story to tell (someday), but for now he will tell you that he uncovered some suppressed tragedies he had not dealt with that put him on that path of divorce. Faced with two attempted suicides, multiple therapists, and multiple moves between two states, Charles overcame the internal battles that secretly haunted him, and he is a better man for facing his fears, doing the work, and overcoming his battles.

During those two years, after the divorce, we barely talked, much less had a civil conversation. While Charles was getting the help he needed, I found strength in friendships and family. I had many conversations with God and learned the value of getting quiet. I found myself hitting the gym to help with stress or taking walks around the RV park, listening to nature, and focusing on moving forward. At first, I wanted to shy away from the world, turn inward, and keep everyone—especially my coworkers— out. No one knew that my world was silently crumbling. The story I told myself was "at work I need to put on my professional hat, keep my shoulders strong, and keep my chin up!" Thank God my coworkers didn't think that way. I lost about 10 pounds within a couple of weeks, and they noticed.

As much as I thought I was keeping it all together, my coworkers saw it. I didn't have to say a word. Beginning with my immediate supervisor, who was fully aware of what I was going through from the moment Charles told me he wanted a divorce, he would walk by my office and simply ask, "Is today a good day, or a bad day?" I would look up from my computer, which I had been absentmindedly staring at for nearly 30 minutes, and shrug my shoulders and shake my head, saying, "Not a good day." No matter if it was 10 a.m. or 1 p.m., he would order me to shut down my computer and go home or somewhere else to think—to grieve. He gave me permission and the space to do that. I will be forever grateful for his kindness and compassion. I would never go home to sit or lie in my grief, though. Again, I "knew" what I needed to do to deal with the stress and depression, from the books I've read to the various training I received in the Army. I needed to exercise to release endorphins and dopamine chemicals in my mind to pull me out of this funk.

Then, the female coworkers that I worked closely with began looking me in the eye and asking, "Are you okay?" or "What's going on?" At first, I lied. I said, "I'm fine! Just working out a lot and I changed my diet—that's why I've lost so much weight," forgetting they were fellow soldiers who had gone through the same training as me. They knew better, and they were genuinely concerned. That's when I learned to let go of trying to carry the weight of the world on my strong shoulders and give the reins to someone else willing to take them. Going through this experience helped me; it taught me that when I became a caregiver, I needed to ask for help.

Both of my sisters, Renée and Karla, were also there for emotional support, offering their shoulders with every call. They each came down to stay a few days with me, reminding me of my own strength. Karla pulled me out of my misery, encouraging me to engage in life and not hide from it by taking me out for dinner and buying me a new outfit. Karla is always well dressed, and after being in the Army for 30 years, my closet needed an over-haul! From Army fatigues, jeans, and T-shirts to more feminine, stylish items with colors other than OD green, or black and brown. Renée was my comforter, and in addition to simply being there, she also knew how to shift my focus. She shared her ideas on business opportunities she wanted to try and got my mind off my troubles by helping me brainstorm. I'm a problem solver, and helping her work through ideas she had was just the medicine I needed to realize I was fully capable of getting through this thing called divorce and overcoming it. All these ladies were my saving grace, my angels that helped carry me through that tough decision about divorce, and they were there, along with my family, during some of my toughest moments when caring for my brother and mother.

They were my tribe.

Find your tribe.

Sooner rather than later.

You never know why you might be going through something challenging now, but in due time, the reasons reveal themselves. How you navigate those challenges are the lessons you are supposed to learn. As heartbreaking as it was to divorce the man of my dreams, my soulmate, the day the divorce was final, I knew in my heart of hearts that it "needed" to happen. Charles asked me to stop the divorce twice. The first time I agreed, but within a week, I knew it needed to continue. There was peace in my heart and in my soul. Had we stopped the divorce, he may have never found the one therapist that helped him discover what he had buried. Charles's PTSD possibly could have reared its ugly head again later had we stayed married.

For me, I may have never experienced the love and compassion of my coworkers, developing the friendships I now have with them, and the closeness with my sisters. I may have never learned to get quiet enough to hear God's voice or recognize the Holy Spirit's nudges, especially the ones that later gave me the comfort and assurance of knowing that caring for my mom and brother was right where I was supposed to be. The divorce had to happen. Also, I believe that Charles and I would not have been able to agree on—much less be prepared to take on—what would be an even greater challenge, which was caring for my brother and mother, had we stayed married.

Protecting Your Loved Ones from the Outside World

In February 2020, my sister-in-law Janice (Marcus's wife) passed away from Alzheimer's. During the funeral, my siblings and I noticed how worn-down Momma looked. Caring for Clint for nearly three years while going through chemotherapy to fight breast cancer that had returned but, in her spine, had taken its toll on her. We had been discussing the possibility of me taking in Clint to care for him and give Mom a break. Seeing her, we began to mentally prepare Mom and told her that by the end of summer, I would come get Clint and move him in with me. I was retired, living alone, while my other siblings were still working regular jobs or caring full time for their grandchildren. Not only did it make sense for me to be Clint's full-time caregiver, but I had been working on developing my relationship with God, and spiritually I felt a calling to it. I felt as though God had given me a clear understanding of how to communicate with Clint and serve as not only a translator to medical personnel but, as I would soon discover, mediator and advocate for both my brother and mother.

I became a volunteer with the Alzheimer's Organization to teach family members about the stages and types of dementia. I also wanted to gain a better understanding of dementia. Being an instructor in the Army, I knew the fastest way to learn is to teach. The day I was to teach my first class in June 2020, I received a phone call from an ER nurse in the small town where Mom and Clint lived. She told me that my mother had been brought in by ambulance for a severe UTI (urinary tract infection) and she was going to be admitted to the hospital but needed someone to pick up Clint. I lived in Tampa, six hours away. I told the nurse I would come but by the time I arrived, it would have been too late to come to the hospital. She told me that they had discovered Clint had a mild UTI, which allowed them to "admit" him as well so he could stay there with Mom. But Clint didn't stay in his room; instead, he sat in the chair next to Mom's bed until I arrived the next day.

I drove up immediately and got to a hotel room. The next morning, I chose to run by Mom's trailer to pick up some of Clint's clothes, check on the animals, and pack up Clint's medications. My intention was to go ahead and move Clint immediately, instead of waiting till fall. While at Mom's, I needed to "freshen up" Clint's clothes and put them in the dryer with a dryer sheet. Mom had Clint's dog, a 120-pound German Shepherd (his other German Shepherd had passed away the year prior), a small dog, and two cats whose litter box she rarely cleaned out. A fact of life growing up with and ashamed to admit, but Mom loved cats, owning close to 10 at one time (if not more). I hated having friends over because of the smell. So, it was necessary to "freshen up" Clint's clothes.

Before I turned on the dryer, something told me to "check the dryer vent!" Mom had an older dryer where the vent was located on the top. I struggled to pull out the nearly 20-inch lint trap due to the amount of lint clinging to it. After tugging on it as hard as I could, it finally came out, revealing about four inches of thick lint (hence my struggle to pull it out). This was a fire hazard waiting to happen! It then occurred to me, not only did Clint need to move in with me, but so did Mom. Our other brother Marcus, who had lived nearby, had since moved to Tennessee. That move left Mom alone and leaning on a community that was aging with her and could not provide the support she needed at age 80. When I arrived at the hospital, I learned that Clint had slept in Mom's room in the chair next to her and refused to leave her side. I also learned that Mom had been delusional due to the UTI. The nurses explained that when someone of Mom's age gets a UTI that goes untreated, it affects them much harder than when someone younger gets a UTI. For example, they can hallucinate, they can struggle to speak or make clear sentences.

When I walked into Mom's room, she looked at me and said, "There you are. I was wondering when you would get here. I talked to you Friday and you told me you were on your way." It was Tuesday morning. I told Mom, "I haven't talked to you in over a week. We never spoke on Friday." She was confused, as the look on her face revealed. She said, "No, that's not right. I wasn't feeling good, and I made Clint lay down with me in my bed so I could keep an eye on him. Then you called me and told me you were on your way." I assured Mom we did not talk, at least not in real life. I pondered the possibility that maybe her guardian angel comforted her in those moments, knowing that I would be coming in a few days.

What I did learn, though, was that she really did make Clint lay down with her, and they stayed in her room all weekend, drinking only water and not eating anything because of her weakness from the UTI. But when Mom and Clint did not show up to church Sunday, the pastor's wife called to check on them early Monday morning.

Something I do love about small towns, especially small churches, is that they check on you when you don't show up. Mom couldn't speak when she answered the phone. As she mumbled, the pastor immediately called 911. Clint had to ride in the back of the ambulance with Mom, which was challenging because Clint didn't seem to understand what was going on, nor could he communicate his emotions and became somewhat combative. At least to others he appeared combative. If you consider the individual, Clint was struggling to articulate words and sentences to relay details of what was going on. Seeing it from that perspective now gives meaning to his behavior. He was frustrated and had no control over what was going on. If *you* could not articulate a cohesive sentence to communicate to the person standing in front of you that your mother was ill and you both had been lying in bed for at least four days with no food, only water, and not sure if the pets were cared for or even let outside to relieve themselves, wouldn't you also get angry and frustrated?

I explained to Mom that it was time for Clint to move in with me and that I would stay until she was released, but Clint would be leaving with me. I told her we were all concerned for her, and I had also decided to move her in with me too. I told her that upon her release, Renée would come get her and she would stay with Renée for a week to recover. After that, Mom would have 30 days to start packing all that she wanted to bring with her to move in with me. We told Mom it was time for her to be taken care of and that she had done enough to help everyone around her. It was time for her to relax. But she didn't like the thought of moving again. She didn't want to leave her home, understandably so. She had found her tribe and made Georgia her home.

She was well-known in her church community and actively participated in church events and gatherings. Her home and land were paid off, and she simply didn't like the idea of packing up her belongings and moving. But she knew she needed to. Marcus was no longer around to help her when she needed it, and now Clint would no longer be there for her to care for. Begrudgingly, she conceded, and in July 2020, I moved Mom down to live with me in Tampa.

Going back to my arrival at the hospital, I found Clint sitting in the chair next to Mom. He looked so tired, wearing a T-shirt, pajama pants, and only socks (no shoes)—he nearly looked catatonic. The nurses tried to get him to eat, but he refused. No one could get him to engage. I squatted down in front of Clint and touched his hand as I began talking to him. "Hey, Clint. It's me, Julie. How are you doing?" He squeezed my hand. This told me he recognized me, but his body language was very tense and stressful. I stood up and kissed him on his forehead, then got directly in front of him so he could see me. I placed my forehead on his forehead and said, "I see you" with a smile. He grinned and mumbled, "I see you." I hugged him, then grabbed his hands and asked him to stand up. He did, and I hugged him again. I walked him over to Momma's bed and asked him to sit on the bed next to Mom. Momma grabbed his hand and arm, stroking it lightly and asking him how he was feeling and if he was hungry. Still feeling a little unsure, he said, "No." I offered him some water and he drank a lot of it. The time came for us to leave. I wanted to get Clint back to the hotel so I could get him bathed and in some fresh clothes.

We loved on Momma and told her we would be back the following day, then walked out of her room. However, as I tried walking Clint down the hallway toward the elevator, he kept pulling back and yelling, "No!" He looked at me with suspicion, as if I was going to hurt him (or that's how I felt)—or maybe he didn't want to leave Momma. I knew I wanted to get him back to the hotel to clean him up, get him to eat, and rest.

I needed to continue to try to move forward by first getting him to the elevator, then to my car, and finally to the hotel. Everything else will fall into place. He just needed to know that Momma was okay and that I was there to help him. I needed to figure out a way to gain his trust somehow.

I firmly locked my arm around his and, speaking very calmly, continued to put one foot in front of the other, pausing as needed to listen to what he was trying to communicate—either with his broken words or his body language. When we reached the elevator, he refused to get in. In my mind I was thinking, what is it? What is it about stepping into this elevator that is making you scared? I continued to talk calmly to Clint and encouraged him that there was no one else on the elevator and it was just the two of us. He struggled to articulate it, but he acted like he saw something in the elevator or was remembering something about it (maybe when they moved him from the ER to the room). I'm not sure what it was, but he was terrified of getting in. He began saying with defeat, "Oh, come on! Come on!" (as if questioning why he had to do this again). I hugged Clint, continuing to assure him he was safe and that I would not let anyone hurt him. I asked if he trusted me. He said "yes." I then asked him to hold my hand and walk with me. We entered the elevator.

Once inside, he was better but still stressed about being in there, at one point even saying, "They're trying to kill me! I know what you're trying to do to me!" I assured him no one was trying to kill him and that we were there to help him. As we stepped out of the elevator to walk toward the lobby doors, he stopped again, pulling away from me and now screaming, "No! No!" I continued to speak calmly to him, asking, "I'm right here, Clint. Do you know who I am?" You could see the constant shifting, back and forth, in his mind of whether to trust or not to trust. A doctor was in her office and heard him screaming. She stepped out to observe what was happening. As Clint continued to yell,

"No!" the doctor stepped forward and asked if I needed help. I put my hand up and said calmly, "No, it's okay." Looking at Clint, I continued to share that our mother was brought into the hospital for a severe UTI and that I think my brother is still worried about her. "I'm taking him home to care for him while she recovers here in the hospital." By that time, Clint had relaxed. As I began to step forward again to leave, Clint willingly walked with me to the car.

Mom was released after a couple of days. I took her back to her trailer, and soon after, Clint and I left for Tampa, suitcase and belongings in hand. A few days after being back in my RV, my eyes to his disease really began to open. I thought back to when I had brought Dad and Clint to stay with me in my RV shortly after Christmas 2019. Dad was 85 and battling his own health problems (Parkinson's—another form of dementia), but Clint was still able to make sentences then. For the most part, anyway. It was like playing charades, with me watching his body language, hand gestures, and facial expressions, then naming one thing after the next until I said the right thing. He would sigh in relief, like "finally!"

Now, he could barely get out a word or two at a time. The disease has progressed in only six months.

These photos were taken on the day I picked up Clint in June 2020 and the day after visiting Mom before her discharge. The last picture was the lint vent from Momma's dryer.

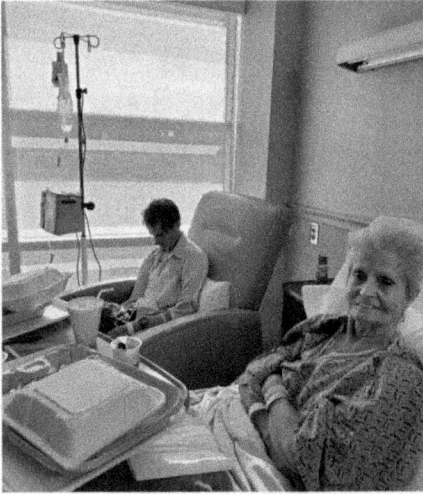

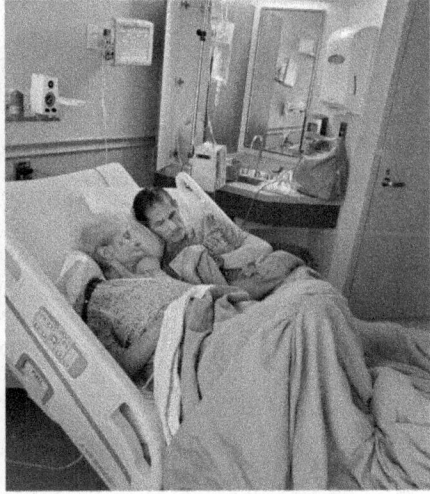

(left) Clint & Mom, Day I arrived to hospital
(right) Mom & Clint, after a day of rest and cleanup, 2020

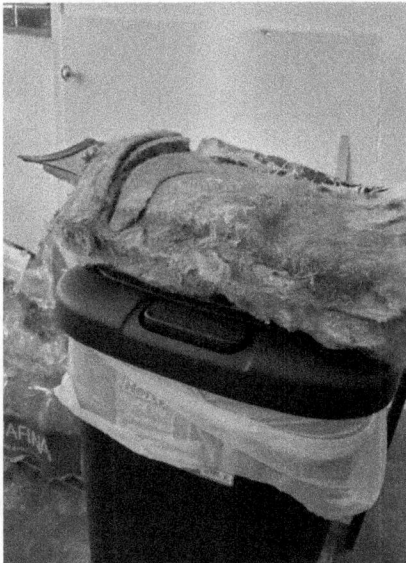

Dryer Lint Trap at Mom's, 2020

Stepping into the Advocate Role

I went through all his medication and wrote out the schedule for each to ensure I kept him on track. One of his medications was in the benzodiazepine family, called Klonopin (a.k.a. clonazepam). The DEA website describes them as follows: "Benzodiazepines are depressants that produce sedation and hypnosis, relieve anxiety, and muscle spasms, and reduce seizures. The most common benzodiazepines are the prescription drugs Valium®, Xanax®, Halcion®, Ativan®, and Klonopin®."

I remember when Clint was still on active duty, working at the Pentagon under the Surgeon General when Xanax first came on the market. He told Dad, "Stay away from Xanax! That is really bad stuff!" I never got the full story of why he thought it was bad, but if Clint had awareness to choose his medications, I doubt he would agree to taking Klonopin. Nonetheless, because anxiety is part of his dementia diagnosis, the doctors had him on it. However, according to the prescription, he is to only take it "as needed" or PRN. So, on his schedule, I wrote "PRN." Behavior-wise, he was doing well.

One day I took him on my golf cart for a ride around the RV park. At one point, he touched my arm and asked me to stop. As he began contemplating his thoughts and struggled to say what was on his mind, he said to me, calmly, "Please kill me. I'm tired of this." I grabbed his hand and said, "No—I'm not going to do that. You are my brother, and I love you."

Another day, he asked me, "Aren't you retired?" I told him I was. He then asked, "But you have a life. Why take care of me? You need to live your life." I told him, "I am! You are my life right now, and I am living it with you. You are my brother, and you need me right now." He sobbed, nodded his head, and said, "Thank you." Then, at another time, he would out of the blue say to me, in a calm and soft tone, "I know what you are doing, and I want to say thank you!" Same words he said that day in the hospital elevator, but now with trust and love. Talk about warming my heart. That was the Clint I knew, and it was confirmation for me that I was right where I needed to be.

The week after Clint moved in with me, Mom, Renée, and my younger brother, Corey, came to my place to celebrate Clint's birthday. He was turning 58 years old. After taking Mom home from the hospital, I brought their smallest dog, Charlie home with me, while Corey took Clint's dog, Tanzer (pronounced "Ten-zer," which means "Dancer" in German). Renée took the two cats, all to lighten Mom's load as she recovered, then prepared to pack up and move in with me. We had a great gathering for Clint's birthday. A few friends from the park came over, and Clint danced a few dances with Renée, me, and Mom. This disease couldn't rob him of his passion for good music and dancing and the love of his family! For that, we were all grateful! I would quickly discover the power of music with someone with FTD.

I've read studies that show how music can brighten up someone with dementia or settle them down when they become agitated. I can attest to the accuracy of those studies, as I was successful in using music as a form of therapy for Clint. There was one time it didn't work, though. It was a few days after his birthday. We had a successful shower (bath) time. Why successful? Another lesson I learned about people with dementia is that when you get them in the tub for bathing, aside from the experience of getting them into the tub and undressed, once they are naked, their internal thermostat is off-kilter, and they perceive excessive cold. Fortunately, because Clint had spent a few days with me a few months earlier, I learned that I needed to *prepare* the bathroom for shower time. This included turning on a small heater and warming up the room (to about 75-80 degrees), having the shower chair ready for him to sit down on, laying out his towel, pajamas, socks, and underwear. We had a great routine in place, and I'd like to believe it was what led to a great "shower time" that night. Unfortunately, things changed in the middle of the night, and maybe it was the calm before the storm.

Clint woke up a little after 3 a.m. and sat up in bed. He was sleeping on the pull-out couch in the living room. I heard him get up, so I went to him and asked if he needed to use the bathroom. He said yes. I followed our normal routine of me taking his hands to help him stand. I then began walking backward to guide him to the stairs. I was wearing my wrist brace, as my carpal tunnel had been acting up. The kitchen counter and sink are within a couple of steps from the pull-out couch, and the moment we stepped in front of the counter, I noticed Clint tightened his grip on my wrists and began pulling back.

At first, I thought maybe he was still asleep and maybe he thought he was losing his balance. So, I reassured him that I had him and secured my grip on his hands. As he tightened his grip on my hands, especially the one with the brace on it, I could feel or sense his whole body tense up and he stopped walking, pulling me toward him instead. I continued to talk to him calmly.

"Clint, it's okay. I got you, but if you keep pulling, you're going to knock me down." But his grip got tighter. "Clint! What's going on? Walk with me. I'm trying to help you up the stairs. Stop pulling!" There was only a nightlight on and the light outside the bathroom was on, so I could see the expressions on his face. He began to grimace as his brain started going into fight-or-flight mode. Clint had this glare in his eyes and didn't know where he was. Suddenly, he saw me as a stranger, someone to fight off. He planted his feet and said, "No." I continued to talk to Clint, telling him, "Clint, it's Julie. If you need to go to the bathroom, I will help you get there, but you're hurting my wrists."

Clint became defensive and strong-armed me, saying, "No! No! You are not! You are a bad man!" I had to switch gears and go into safety mode to ensure Clint's safety. Clint began pushing me. I guided that push toward the stairs to get him to where there was better lighting, then tripped walking up the stairs backward. He had a death grip on my arms by this point. I was able to get him into the bathroom, where he pinned me against the wall. Mind you, we were in an RV, where the bathroom barely has enough room for a sink, toilet, and stand-up shower. I had left my curling iron out on the sink and suddenly saw it as a potential weapon. I didn't want him to find it.

As a reminder, he could barely see (no peripheral vision), and although he still struggled to form sentences, in this state of mind, he was able to say what he needed to. I got him to release me enough to grab the curling iron and throw it under the cabinet. By then, he slipped by me, facing the sink and the mirror, and began pushing on the mirror and the adjacent cabinet and making this loud humming noise. It was so loud I was afraid if anyone was outside, they would hear him. It was nearly 4 a.m., so it was very quiet in the RV park. You could hear someone's TV if it was on.

He remained in this state for 20 or 30 minutes. I talked to him. I sang to him, "Jesus loves me, this I know" because Renée would often sing it to him. I tried placing a wet towel on the back of his neck, reading scripture to ward off any demonic presence, and caressing his head. His body was so rigid.

Finally, he ended up following me down the stairs (stumbled), knocking over the vacuum cleaner and wiping anything sitting on the kitchen counter onto the floor, as if he were coming after me. It was at this point that I called 911. I immediately told them all the important information: this is my brother, and he has dementia. The last thing I needed was cops to roll up there trying to tackle him and put handcuffs on him. Clint could hear me on the phone as his anxiety level continued to rise. He went from the kitchen counter to the coffee counter and began knocking those items onto the floor. I got him to stop just before the coffee pot went tumbling with everything else. While I'm still on the phone with 911, Clint slapped me, then started yelling that "a man put his dick up my"—then slapped his bottom. This surprised me just as much as it is surprising you right now, reading it. I had no idea what he was talking about and wondered if this could possibly be a childhood memory, a terrible childhood memory.

When the police arrived, I let them in, and they kept their distance while I explained the details of all that happened within the last hour. They also tried talking to Clint calmly and without going near him. I even called Mom to ask for her help and to see if she could not only talk him down from this episode, maybe hearing her voice would settle him—but also to see if she had experienced this with him. If so, how did she handle it? Mom tried talking to Clint. It wasn't immediate, but he did begin to settle after maybe another 20 or 30 minutes.

Mom asked if I had given Clint his Klonopin. I told her that he hadn't "needed" it, and this was the first time he had reacted like this. He was in no state to take any medications willingly. An ambulance arrived, and the EMTs were able to help me walk Clint out to the gurney, where he cooperated, and they were able to get him loaded into the ambulance. I gave them his ID and followed them to the hospital. Unfortunately, on the trip, Clint became combative again, and they gave him a shot of something in the benzodiazepine family to sedate him.

Once at the ER, as I was walking into the room, they had just rolled him into, Clint had a death grip on the rails of the gurney and was trying to get up off the bed. The two security guards and three or four nurses trying to hold him down said he was very strong. The nurses also gave him a spray up his nose to further calm him. It took about 15 or 20 minutes for all the medication to kick in. We stayed in the ER for nearly six hours before Clint was finally admitted.

After a phone call to the hospital administrator, they allowed me to stay with him in his hospital room. As a reminder, this was 2020 and COVID was in full swing. At first, the doctors were *not* going to allow me to stay with him "because" of COVID conditions. I told them he did not have COVID and that was not why he was there. They tried to give me the "hospital protocol" crap, but I did not accept that response. I *demanded* to speak with the hospital administrator. I reminded the doctors that, although Clint exhibited combative behavior, he had a diagnosis of frontotemporal dementia, no peripheral vision, and was unable to communicate to hospital staff his needs, much less the mental clarity to legally sign any paperwork.

I told them they needed me to act as a go-between: I was his voice, his advocate for being able to speak about what was best for his care and in his best interest. I carried with me his power of attorney and healthcare surrogate paperwork and showed it to the doctor. I told him I did not give him permission to administer any medications or care unless I was by his side. The hospital administrator gave the approval, and I slept on the hospital recliner next to Clint's bed. It wasn't until 9 p.m. that the doctors decided to give him a new anxiety pill. It left him groggy until 2 p.m. the following day. He started coming out of it, but because of that medication, he could barely stand, much less walk. The prognosis given was that Clint needed to see a psychiatrist to manage his medication and treat his anxiety.

I later learned that Mom had been giving Clint his Klonopin medication daily. She had been so overwhelmed with caring for him, two dogs, two cats, and managing her own cancer treatment that she apparently went on autopilot and stopped taking the time to read the actual prescription bottle. She got into the habit of giving him what she thought he was supposed to take. Taking that into consideration, he had been under my care for about seven days with no Klonopin. His psychiatrist and I came to the determination that what most likely happened was he was having withdrawals and that caused the psychotic episode. I shared with the psychiatrist that I would prefer to get him back to taking such types of medication on a PRN basis, along with removing any other medications that weren't pertinent to his disease. The psychiatrist agreed and worked with me to adjust his medications, tapering off what was no longer needed or necessary.

July soon rolled around, and with the help of my sisters, Karla and Renée, and our youngest brother, Corey, Mom moved in. I placed my RV up for sale and rented a three-bedroom apartment just across the street from the church I attended. Mom stayed at the apartment by herself for the first few weeks while I took a slower transition with Clint in moving him over. He and I would "go visit Mom" then go "home" to sleep. Continuing to learn more about people with FTD and other types of dementia, the studies stressed the importance of a slow transition when needing to move them from one home to another—possibly another factor in Clint's psychotic episode the previous month.

I reached out to the Alzheimer's hotline to share my experience and asked if there was anything more I could've done. One suggestion had to do with the lighting in the RV. They shared that many people with dementia who have vision problems tend to see shadows in dim light. Therefore, I should ensure that a regular light is always on for when they wake up in the middle of the night. Another suggestion was to ease them into a new home. So, once Mom arrived, we would just go "visit." That eventually turned into spending the night (sleepover), then fully moving in and explaining, "This is your room, your bed, our kitchen, and we all live together." By that September, I sold my RV as Clint settled into his new living arrangement.

Retired, divorced, and a full-time caregiver for two family members, believe it or not, I felt content. I had tried the dating scene soon after the divorce, but it wasn't what I wanted. I did not have the emotional energy to deal with an intimate relationship. My time and energy were needed to care for my brother and mother, and I was okay with that. I did have some challenges caring for Clint, and my church provided me with the spiritual support—and sometimes the physical support—I needed.

Mom and Clint both really enjoyed Sunday services, Bible studies, and prayer night, and Clint especially enjoyed the music. He would place his hands on the chair in front of him and start tap-tap-tapping (drumming) with the rhythm of the songs. Every little sign of "Clint" that showed through warmed our hearts and put a big smile on Mom's face. Seeing her son living with this disease was heartbreaking. Occasionally, I would catch a tear in her eyes. Sometimes they were tears of joy and sometimes of sadness. Mom struggled with expressing her emotions. I believe in her mind she needed to stay strong. And strong, she absolutely was.

The three of us slowly settled into a routine, of sorts. It took me a few weeks to find my rhythm: navigating each of their doctors, scheduling their appointments (ensuring there was no overlap), and ensuring my own health needs were being taken care of. I found myself at first forgetting to write down an appointment (my own) and then would get the call of "Are you still coming to your appointment?" The first two times this happened, being the perfectionist I am, I literally cried because I dropped the ball. No one blamed me. I blamed myself, and I can be hard on myself. A part of me thought that maybe I could get a job, so I tried interviewing for a few roles that were remote. I believe my guardian angels watched out for me because they knew what was coming down the pike and blocked each of those interviews from either happening or succeeding (I bombed on a couple). Another shift in Clint's disease was on the immediate horizon.

The apartment complex had a large pond that we could take walks around. A few times a week, the three of us would take walks just to get some fresh air and so Clint could get some exercise. I quickly learned to communicate with Clint, at least by deciphering his behavior and body language. Mostly I would ask him yes or no questions and he could respond appropriately. Clint began pacing throughout the apartment and would suddenly drop to his knees and begin patting the floor, almost like he was hammering but with his hand. Mom and I would just watch. After a few minutes, I would ask him, "Whatcha doing, Clint?" He would, very clearly, say, "I'm piddling." That could last anywhere from 5 minutes to 15 minutes. I would just observe him, making sure he didn't bump into anything or knock anything over.

There were times he would walk around the apartment, touching countertops or cabinets, smoothing them down with his hands. Again, I would curiously ask, "Hey, Clint! Whatcha doing?" The expression on his face would be one of "this is important," like he was working. He often would tell me, "This is a boat!" I could never definitively figure that one out, but I'm sure it had something to do with a boat he used to own.

With him struggling to articulate his needs, I would often ask him if he needed to go to the bathroom. Like a child, he would become agitated or frustrated about something. After asking a few questions, it would finally click, and I would say, "Do you need to go pee?" With a sigh of relief, he would nod his head and sometimes get the word "Yes" out. He did struggle with constipation, and whenever he needed to go poop, his agitation would increase significantly, but then he would start rambling the word "Four-Four-Four," repeatedly. It took some time, but I eventually began connecting this behavior and those words to him needing to go poop. The best I could make of all that was he used to play golf. When you get relief from a good poop, what better thing to say than "FOUR!!!!!"

He began waking up in the middle of the night. When I took him to the bathroom, I would have him sit down to urinate. His vision had gotten worse, and it no longer made sense for him to try and "aim." But in his mind, he knew he was a man and knew that a man stands up. When he began waking in the middle of the night, his room was directly across from the bathroom. We kept the bathroom light on all night. He would make his way to the door of the bathroom and do his thing, then go back to bed. I would find "the surprise," if Mom didn't first when she would get up in the middle of the night to go to the bathroom (oops!). I needed to find a way to have him set off an alarm to let me know he was out of bed. So, I would take three or four empty water bottles and lay them across the threshold of his bedroom door. It worked like a charm! He would get up and would inevitably kick the water bottles, sending them across the tile floors. I was a light sleeper (like a mother with a sick child) and it would wake me immediately. I eventually purchased a bed alarm that slid under the mattress. They were pressure sensitive, so the minute he got off the bed, the alarm would go off. I also bought a nanny camera to keep an eye on him that way. I would help him to the bathroom, then put him back in bed.

One day, around the middle of August 2020, after I got home from grocery shopping, I came in to find Clint being fussy with Mom. She was trying to calm him down but didn't understand what he was trying to say. I tried asking him what was going on, but he was just jabbering away, so I kept putting away groceries. At one point he said, "That's okay, you'll see." I heard him but kept putting away the groceries with Mom's help. Mom then went to her room, and I turned my back for maybe five minutes. The next thing I knew, Clint was out the door. He ran out past the pond and behind the apartment complex. By the time I caught up with him, I had pulled my calf muscle and was in a lot of pain, not to mention out of breath. I grabbed his hand and told him to come back to the apartment. Honestly, I lost my composure and did everything you're not supposed to do. He was yelling and fussing, and I yelled back. At this point it was a brother-and-sister argument! I began walking at a fast pace with him in tow, having no compassion or desire to placate or pacify him. At that moment in time, he was acting like a child. He basically said he was tired of everything and tired of being inside all day. I asked him if he wanted to get some exercise, and he said "Yes!"

So, I said, "Okay…let's go for a jog" (my calf muscle relaxed enough to jog). We jogged back to the apartment with my arm interlocked with his. I began talking to him like a drill instructor (we were both in the military, so I knew he would get it). He got a smile on his face. I got him back to the apartment, and he started arguing again. He kept saying that others and I were making fun of him, saying things that weren't true, then accused me of "falling away," said he saw me and began describing something like "a balloon." I had no clue what he was talking about. I finished with the groceries, made dinner, and nothing more was said.

His early morning trips to the bathroom continued. We met with his psychiatrist, and he put him on medicine to help slow down his urge to pee throughout the night. Over the next two months, I began noticing Clint becoming more and more agitated, especially in the evening. His doctor suggested he had something called "sundowners." The Mayo Clinic describes it like this: "The term 'sundowning' refers to a state of confusion occurring in the late afternoon and lasting into the night. Sundowning can cause different behaviors, such as confusion, anxiety, aggression, or ignoring directions. Sundowning can also lead to pacing or wandering." https://www.mayoclinic.org/diseases-conditions/alzheimers-disease/expert-answers/sundowning/faq-20058511#:~:text=The%20term%20%22sundowning%22%20refers%20to,Sundowning%20isn't%20a%20disease.

Soon after starting this medication, Clint began getting up in the middle of the night and pacing, walking around the apartment, thinking he needed to leave or go somewhere. Working with his psychiatrist, we had begun tapering him off some of the medications he no longer needed and starting him on a new one. But Clint went into full-blown insomnia a week or so later. He wasn't sleeping and could not—would not—go to bed. It was as though he was on speed. He would go to bed on time, sleep for about two hours, then wake up for three or four hours. I would sit with him, walk with him, and often lie next to him in his bed, rubbing his back or forehead, trying to calm him to go to sleep. Sometimes it worked; sometimes, no sooner would I leave his room, he would pop right back up and the cycle would start all over again. This lasted for nearly 30 days. I was barely functioning on two or three hours of sleep a night! I felt as though I would go insane. I called the doctors to find out what was wrong and how to get him to sleep. He would be up all night, and during the day, he started having more and more agitation, sometimes screaming so loud I was waiting for a neighbor to call the police.

The one thing I did find to console him was classical piano music. I like to listen to Pandora and decided to install the app on the smart TV. I would play artists like Philip Wesley or Yiruma. I was somewhat surprised—and elated—the first time I put on this music during one of his episodes. His whole body softened, the tension in his face relaxed, and he would go dead silent, often falling asleep or just drifting off into a meditative gaze. I vaguely remembered hearing about studies being done with dementia patients and the effects of listening to music. Then I remembered my experience with my sister-in-law, Janice. When Janice's Alzheimer's began to progress, I experimented with this theory about music. I put earbuds in her ears and began to play her favorite Christian songs whenever her anxiety levels would

begin to rise. It was like watching a light turn on! Her face bright-
ened, her eyes went wide, and she started dancing in her seat and
singing every word to the song being played. Our hearts just
melted as we all teared up. There was Janice.

I tried different genres of music with Clint. The soft classical
piano music was best for tempering his anxiety, while hip-hop,
disco music, and contemporary Christian music got him on his
feet and dancing again, just like the Clint, we knew him to be. I
eventually found an actual study that AFTD wrote about on their
website on how effective music can be with dementia patients. It
is a great read and brought me comfort knowing that I was on
the right track. You can read it here (https://www.the-
aftd.org/posts/1ftd-in-the-news/bbc-music-therapy-people-
with-dementia/).

I recently learned that our brains respond to classical music
through the release of dopamine. I found the following study
about how listening to classical music can help with health issues
such as lowering blood pressure, improving focus, and reducing
anxiety.

Stress and anxiety relief
Neurologist Dr. Corey Schneck found that classical music helps
relieve anxiety. More and more studies are finding that music
helps lower cortisol levels, which are associated with stress. A
post by Lottoland on how music is good for your health states
that it also increases blood flow by 26%, laughter by 16%, and
relaxation by 11%. Indeed, research published in *Complementary
Therapies in Clinical Practice* studied 180 patients and found that

listening to natural sounds, classical Turkish, or Western music helped reduce anxiety by lowering cortisol levels, blood pressure, and heart rate. While they all led to positive attributes, the classical Turkish music proved to be the most effective in stress and anxiety relief.

https://myscena.org/newswire/the-science-behind-why-classical-music-is-good-for-mental-health/

Nonetheless, after nearly three weeks of no sleep, I continued to reach out to his neurologists, his psychiatrist, and his primary care physician at the VA clinic, begging and pleading for help. The neurologist, whom I thought was his "dementia" doctor, said, "He has a psychiatric problem; you need to call them." The psychiatrist's assistant would always take my calls, and eventually she recommended taking him to an ER so they could admit him. She suggested that if Clint was becoming combative, I needed to seek help by starting with the ER. Once in the ER, they would decide to admit him under the Baker Act. However, the more I called, the more I heard that the state of Florida would not "Baker Act" a dementia patient. "SO, WHAT AM I SUPPOSED TO DO?" Remember, I was trying to function on two hours of sleep for over three weeks. I was becoming delirious (at least I felt like I was). I was exhausted, defeated, and angry that there was no system or process in place to assist family members in caring for someone with dementia. "Aren't you the doctors? Aren't you the ones trained in this stuff? What the HELL am I supposed to do?" Clint would push and grab your arm. Mom would sometimes try to help, and I would have to yell at her to step away to avoid her being hurt. She was 5 feet 2 inches, about

120 pounds, and still battling cancer. Clint was very strong, and as much as I knew he would never hurt his mother, the possibility was there. I couldn't keep them both safe, so I would have her step away. Sometimes I would have to wrestle Clint to the ground—not aggressively, just guide him down—to disorient him, change his posture by getting him to lay flat on his back, and interrupt the agitation pattern. I would immediately turn on Pandora and start playing Philip Wesley music. Clint would be humming in an agitated way, but after about 10 minutes, he would start to calm down. I was able to talk to him calmly and ask if he was ready to get up. He would say yes, I would help him up and guide him over to the couch, where he would sit peacefully, listening to the music. Every single day and night, this cycle would be repeated. I was beyond exhausted.

By the middle of November, around 8 p.m., I drove Clint to the VA clinic ER. Once we got into a room, the medicine that I had given him while we were in the waiting room started to kick in and he relaxed. The ER doctor came in to ask questions and find out what had been going on. He called in a psychiatrist to discuss options to assist Clint with getting some sleep. The psychiatrist explained about not being able to Baker Act him due to his dementia, and we discussed possible medications that he could take. She left to input her notes into the system, and we were waiting to be released from the ER. The ER doctor returned, however, as they still needed to get a CT of Clint, as was protocol. An x-ray technician came in to get Clint to roll him just down the hall for the CT scan (I could see the room from where we were). Within a few minutes, I could hear a commotion going on down the hallway. I walked down, and the technician and the nurse were struggling to get Clint to lay down for the CT. I stood there patiently observing, allowing them to do what they needed to do, until the nurse looked at me and said, "This isn't going to work." I said, "Okay, do you want to just bring him back to the room?" The nurse moved Clint out of the CT room. Clint was becoming more restless, trying to get off the gurney. The nurse was nervous and confused and not sure what to do. I knew exactly what I needed to do. I looked at the nurse square in his eyes and said, "I can handle him, but I need to…" I didn't finish my sentence or ask permission. I jumped up on top of the gurney, straddled Clint, and held down his shoulders. I got directly in front of Clint (remember, he had no peripheral vision, so I needed to be directly in front of him for him to see me) and calmly started talking to him. "Clint, it's Julie. You're okay, but I need you to breathe. Take a deep breath for me, Clint. Look at me, listen to my voice, and breathe." As I sat straddled on the gurney, talking and holding Clint down, the nurse rolled us down the hallway and back into the room. We rolled right past the small room where the doctors sat to type up or dictate their notes, and the ER doctor looked up in amazement to see me on top of the gurney. He jumped up and followed us into the room. The ER doctor then asked, "Is this what you have been dealing with?" I said, "Yes! Every single night for the past month." He ordered the nurse to get a cocktail of sedatives and told me, "We are admitting him tonight. You need to get some rest; we'll take it from here." I wanted to stay with him, but "COVID." It was the VA, Clint was being admitted to the psychiatric ward, and they had a strict policy of no visitors allowed. I wrote out on a napkin everything I wanted his team of nurses and doctors to know: "He goes by his middle name, 'Clint.' Please call him Clint." Also, "Classical piano music calms him. Look up artists like Philip Wesley, Yiruma, or Denise Young." I made sure they had my number and pleaded that they would call me, no matter the time of day, if they had any difficulty communicating with him. That was the beginning of the discovery that benzodiazepines needed to be removed from his prescription lists.

You know your loved one, and while medical personnel have skill and training, they lack the intimate knowledge you have. Ask questions, take notes, and, once you have a picture, you may have to lay it out for the doctors. Multiple times, sadly.

I went home and straight to bed, only to be awakened by the nursing staff calling me with questions. Questions that were answered on the napkin I taped on his pillow before leaving but were not read or shared by the nurses. They had their routine. This was part of my frustration with medical staff. They reinvent the wheel with every patient by going through a discovery process to learn how to best care for the patient in front of them. From a process improvement perspective, this wastes a lot of time, and it's the patient that suffers. "I left you instructions on how best to communicate and accommodate Clint's needs; you did not read it!" No, that was not a question; it was a direct statement! "Breathe, Julie…." I reminded myself of my tired, restless state.

I did a reset and calmly explained what the nurses needed to do. She looked around and eventually found the napkin I had written notes on. She was thankful to see the information and changed the TV to a music station immediately, playing classical music. They also changed his name on the whiteboard for the next shift to see. Clint was named after our father, so his first name was Ralph but went by his middle name, Clinton (or Clint). After day two, I finally heard from the doctor overseeing Clint's care. He called me to find out what my intentions were. I didn't understand the question. He explained that Clint was in a prime position to be transferred to a nursing home, or did I plan to bring him home. I hesitated. Am I? Am I ready for him to go into a nursing home? It's not what he wants. It's not what Momma wants. What do I do? I told the doctor my intention was to bring him home and asked if they had figured out a way to help him sleep. The doctor stated they had been giving him a sedative, which would be stopped once he was released, and that if I didn't want to have him "placed" [in a home], then he would be released the following day. The doctor didn't answer my question, not quite. I reminded him, "You've given him a sedative to calm him while he's there, but I won't have those cocktails to give him once he is home. What is the plan moving forward?" The doctor seemed unsure, as if waiting for me to give him a possible solution. Once again, I was baffled at what I was experiencing. In my head, I'm screaming, "Aren't YOU the doctor here? What the HELL am I supposed to figure out here?" I asked the doctor to go over all the medications Clint was currently taking. They had Clint on the following medications: Valproic acid (250mg) 2x/day-a mood stabilizer, Memantine (5mg, 2x/day), Clonazepam (1/2 a pill), Melatonin, and Haldol, an antipsychotic

(PRN). He had been on Seroquel upon arrival, but they were able to ween him off it, then Mirtazapine at bedtime. I did not get a plan of action for when Clint got released.

Clint remained at the VA for a total of three nights. When I picked him up, he was so drugged he could barely stand, much less walk from the wheelchair to my car. It took about two days for the Haldol medication to completely get out of his system. However, the side effects had left their mark. I would venture to say that Clint became worse than before he was admitted to the VA. The insomnia not only continued, but the agitation increased, along with the hallucinations. I had been advised by a friend that I should reach out to the social worker at the hospital for assistance on what to do next. I did, and she explained that if I was ready to have Clint placed in a nursing home, I was going to have a lot of difficulty finding a facility to accept him, because he now had a record of being combative. I felt stuck, lost, and abandoned. If not for my family and friends' words of encouragement and my church's support, I could have easily found myself in a psychiatric ward. But I refused to allow that to happen. Clint needed me. Momma needed me. My kids still needed me to be present (in the moment) whenever they called. "Keep it together, Julie," I would remind myself. I would stand in a hot shower, the water just pouring over me as I held the walls, crying, praying for more strength than I thought I had.

I couldn't work out, which is a natural stress reliever. I wasn't sleeping, I had a shoulder injury that was getting worse as caring for Clint became more physical. I needed rotator cuff surgery, and my carpal tunnel continued to flare up. I needed help, and where I thought it would come from, where I expected it to come from, fell way short of that expectation. I called my sisters often, if nothing else, to simply release tension by expressing my frustration and exhaustion. They lived four hours away and had their own families to manage or worked 40 to 60 hours a week. But they would listen and console the best they could.

In less than ten days after coming home from the VA hospital (just before Thanksgiving) and after reaching out to another social worker at a local hospital, I once again took Clint to the ER shortly before lunch, but this time at a non-VA hospital. Clint's anxiety and agitation were so high that I called the ER ahead of time to let them know we were on our way. I wanted to learn their process to mitigate any added trauma of Clint walking into another ER room. They met me in the car and helped me get him into a wheelchair so I could park. I came in and took Clint through the check-in process and fortunately did not have to wait long before they took him back. Once in an ER room, they immediately gave him an Ativan shot at about 1:35 p.m. They said it would take effect within fifteen minutes. By 2:00 p.m., nothing. A second shot was given at 2:15 p.m. I sat with Clint, talking to him to try to get him to settle down. His arms were flailing, and he was moaning and yelling. I was combing through my mind of how to solve this problem. Nothing was coming to mind. The nurses were approaching a shift change, which meant I was on my own until the next string came in to read his chart and get spun up on what was going on. It may have been close to 4:00 p.m. when the new nurse came in for an update. I asked to speak with a doctor, and they didn't know when that would happen. A third Ativan shot was soon given, as Clint was still not settled. I kept pacing back and forth between Clint and the hallway. When a nurse came, they would close the door behind them when they left the room. I would open it because I didn't want them to forget we were in there and they needed to see and hear Clint's outburst or humming.

The staff seemed to be so nonchalant about the patients on the floor and appeared to be taking their time going through charts and chatting with each other. I wanted to shake them and yell, "Hello! Do you not hear my brother! Why isn't anyone coming in here?" Finally, around 6:00 p.m., five and a half hours after arriving at the ER, a psychiatrist came in to evaluate Clint. We discussed "Baker Acting" him to have him admitted to the psych ward, but at a different hospital. I still wasn't clear on the process. Nothing made sense to me. Another two hours went by, and I was hanging on by a thread. I walked through the halls, looking for a nurse to talk to and find out what was going on—why was he not being moved to this other hospital? His nurse came in, and I sort of unloaded (more like, unleashed the Kraken) on her. She was so very patient—listened to every word I said. Then quietly walked over, put her hand on my shoulder, and gently explained what we were waiting for, why we were waiting: for the other hospital to call and let them know if a bed was open and ready for Clint to be moved. She said she would call them directly to see what she could find out. Within five minutes, she returned to say that a bed had just come open. That then gave her the authority to call for transportation. She noted that Clint was sleeping at this point and that they would take care of Clint.

She basically gave me permission to leave so I could go home and rest. She may not have said all those things, but her actions did. It was at that moment I fell over onto Clint's bed and began sobbing and apologizing for yelling at her. Also in that moment, I felt "released" to leave. I did, crawling into bed as soon as I got home. I got a call from the nursing staff at 6 a.m. the next morning, letting me know that Clint was en route to the other hospital's psych ward and providing me with names and numbers to reach his team. I finally felt as though Clint was in the right place —a place where the staff was very familiar with and trained for dementia patients and knew exactly how to manage his behavior. However, because he was being held under the Baker Act, he must go through a hearing with a judge before discharge to decide if he is ready to be released back home and safe to himself and others or if he must stay. It all depended on how well his medications were adjusted and calmed him. They did get his medication leveled out, and he returned home. However, from that point forward, I made sure to tell every one of his doctors to note in his records to never administer any drug in the benzodiazepine family again.

Experts will tell you not to forget to take care of yourself, and I had. Every part of my being—physically, mentally, and emotionally—was caring for Clint. It was taking a toll on my mind and body. For these reasons, I was still not dating anyone. I barely had the energy to care for Clint, much less put any into a relationship. There was someone who was helping me with Clint that very much wanted a more intimate relationship, but I didn't have the energy to give and let him know. Not to mention, my heart still belonged to Charles, even though we were no longer on speaking terms.

I think it was around Christmas that our daughter informed the family she was expecting her first child. She held a Zoom call, and that was the first time I had seen Charles in over a year. Once again, I was smitten but kept it to myself until after the grand-baby was born in 2021. I invited Charles to drop by to visit Clint and Mom and then go to dinner and talk. Maybe it was the wine, but we kissed that night, and once again, it was as if the clouds parted, and the heavenly choir began singing. I felt like a teenage girl being kissed for the first time. Charles and I began texting and calling each other regularly. It was nice to step away from the caregiver role, even if for just a few moments a day to receive those texts. It gave me something to look forward to and, if nothing else, provided me with a short mental break.

I bought a house closer to Jacksonville to be near family and get Clint into an assisted living facility. At first, I thought it was a great place to care for his needs —until I began seeing how he was being cared for.

Fortunately, Clint had a guardian angel who didn't work on his floor. When she discovered how he was being cared for, she would check on him during her breaks, cleaning up his room and bathroom (finding feces or urine on the floor) or simply changing his diaper and clothes that were left soiled. Clint could not artic-ulate his needs (usually to go to the bathroom or drink water), so he would yell out. When no one answered him, he would get out of his wheelchair and try to walk to the bathroom on his own.

Unfortunately, he couldn't see very well and would end up falling after a few steps. He would get frustrated when the staff would get him up and put him back in his chair. The staff viewed this behavior as "being combative." After the first few times of this happening, they got approval from the in-house nurse practitioner to administer Seroquel "as needed." This went on for a few weeks; however, their interpretation of "as needed" became more "routine" than "as needed" to quiet him down and do as they say and to force him into their routine of getting things done and managing all the patients on his floor. The problem was, when he would start coming down from the Seroquel, there were side effects of increased agitation and anxiety. It became a vicious circle.

Within the first month, one of Clint's caregivers caught me as I came in to visit one morning. They didn't know I was coming, and I was there early. When she saw me, she looked frustrated and proceeded to demonstrate her frustration with Clint's behavior. She wanted to show me how uncooperative Clint was when she tried to give him a bath. I was just curious enough to allow her to demonstrate and observe what exactly Clint was experiencing. So, I said, "Sure, let's see." Clint was still asleep when we both walked into his room. He was on his side, facing away from us, toward the wall. The caregiver began talking to Clint as we walked in, to get him to start waking up. She had a naturally loud and commanding voice, not one I would've used, and I knew not one to which Clint responded very well. But I remained silent. "Hey, Clint! It's time to wake up." She put her hands on his shoulder and arm and pulled him to get him to roll to his back, without warning. I recognized it for what it was: she scared Clint, shocking him out of a deep sleep. What do you think his reaction was? His arms and legs began to flail, and he began to yell out.

A second caregiver came in to assist with getting Clint up and ready for a bath. They immediately began removing Clint's clothes while he was still in this shocked state of mind, talking very loudly to him to tell him it was time to take a bath and to calm down. They stripped him naked, then put him in the wheelchair to move him to the bathroom. They put him in the shower chair, and the second girl left, leaving just me and the first caregiver. She turned on the shower wand and allowed it to warm up. All while, Clint was still yelling and trying to get out of the shower chair. The caregiver spoke even louder, yelling at Clint to stay seated and let her clean him up. I was standing there watching because I wanted her to show me her behavior more than I wanted to see his behavior. It wasn't five minutes, and I stopped her. I didn't get into a debate with her, as it would not have served Clint at that moment. But I did ask her, "Why don't you change your approach? Here, let me help you." Clint didn't even know I was there until I opened my mouth. I began talking to Clint in a quiet and calm voice to settle him, and he settled down quickly. I more or less took over giving him a bath.

I explained to her briefly that she needed to take her time with him, to which she quickly retorted, "I don't have time! I have 10 other patients I need to take care of!" It was at that moment I chose to stop talking to her, realizing it wasn't really her fault. It was management's fault for implementing such a strict schedule and deferring to that requirement at the detriment of the patients' care.

I cut to the chase and walked straight into the director's office after my visit with Clint. I expressed my concerns and shared what had happened. I also told him I was not seeking to file a grievance against the caregiver. I told him my grievance was with him and every person in charge of the caregivers. He talked a good game and said he empathized with me, if not agreed or understood my position. He still shifted blame to the caregiver. From that point forward, I stayed on my toes, watching their every move.

I had removed Clint from that facility just four months after admitting him. He wasn't there for 30 days and was already admitted to the ER for dehydration. Never, in either mine or Mom's care, had Clint ever been found to be dehydrated. As I told the facility on their intake form, he loves water —lots and lots of it. Give him as much as he wants. Soon after arriving at the ER, he had a seizure that was brought on from dehydration. I never had that issue while caring for him because I knew how much water he would drink. He loved water, and they were not giving him enough. I later learned they would give him tea or lemonade or, worse, Kool-Aid.

I immediately called the ER to speak with the attending nurse and/or physician to give them some background information on his diagnosis. Thank goodness I did! Once I shared with the team that he had FTD and was unable to communicate his needs, that insight completely changed their perspective. Because Clint had a seizure in the ER, they wanted to give him seizure medication, but only because they thought he had a history of seizures and thought he was supposed to be on it. I told them "NO!" He does not have a history of seizures. He is dehydrated and this was a one-time event. DO NOT add to his list of medications that will only cause more side effects. He needs fluids! Please give him fluids and nothing else. Clint was there alone. No one from the facility was there to guide the ER staff on how to communicate with Clint.

EMS brought him in, handed over a report from the facility stating he had a fever and fell and was disoriented. Now, just think about that for a moment. If you were the ER doctor and given that same information, how would you proceed? They can only pass judgment on the "scenario" presented to them, in that moment of time, to decide on what to do next. I was not about to allow that to happen, hence why I had called to speak with the doctor as soon as I was notified by the facility that Clint was on his way to the ER.

I then drove to the ER to be with him. Renée met me there. She lived about 10 minutes from the hospital. He was calm and relaxed, smiling to see us there. Even drumming out "paradiddles" with Renée. It's an exercise that drummers do when first learning to play drums, and he taught Renée how to do them many years prior. We then called Marcus—and Clint loved hearing Marcus's voice. Clint was admitted for dehydration for one night, then released back to the facility.

I would go through this exercise of Clint being admitted to the ER three more times over the next three months: twice for falling (getting out of his chair when ignored) and the third and last time for being "combative." It was that last time that drove the need to remove him from that facility. Mom and I visited Clint that morning, then ran to the grocery store. As we walked into the house, the director of nursing (DON) called me to let me know that they were struggling to get Clint to settle down. She asked if I would come back to the facility to assist. I said I would and headed that way.

I was one block from the facility when she called again, stating that the nurse practitioner had made the decision to send Clint to the ER for evaluation and the ambulance had just left. I drove past the facility and went straight to the ER. I walked into Clint's room, and he laid there peaceful and calm as he slept, because they had given him an "extra" dose of Seroquel. I sat with him for about an hour before the doctor came in. He asked why Clint was there. I told him about my conversation with the director of nursing and that he was there for "evaluation." The doctor then asked me if I thought Clint looked to be in any distress, to which I replied, "No, he seems very relaxed." Clint was awake at this point and aware of mine and the doctor's presence. The doctor observed me interacting with Clint and wrote in his chart that Clint was okay. The doctor asked me if I was taking him home or if he would be returning to the facility. I told him he was a resident at the assisted living facility and if he was released, that's where he needed to go.

It took about three hours for transportation (an ambulance) to arrive. Once there, I shared with them what I share with each medical staff member we encounter: "He goes by Clint. Please call him Clint. If for some reason he gets agitated, pull your phone out and play music by Philip Wesley or Yiruma." The EMTs *loved* having this information! They were relieved that I was there to share that with them. They rolled him out, and I left. It was about 10 p.m. at this point. I was almost home when I got a phone call from one of the EMTs.

"Hi, Ms. Julie, this is one of the paramedics who just picked up your brother. We are at the facility, and the night nurse is re-fusing to take Clint back. She is telling us that he is no longer a resident at their facility."

My whole body tensed up. My heart began to race, and my face was flushed with heat. I hit my brakes and yelled, "What?!" I said, "He *is* a resident. They were the ones who called the am-bulance to take him to the ER. I want to talk to that nurse." The EMT handed his phone to the night nurse. Just as rude as anyone could possibly be, she did not give me a word edgewise and ad-amantly told me, "Mr. Prescott is no longer a resident here. You spoke to the director of nursing (DON) earlier today, so you know what's going on." I acknowledged speaking with the DON once at the hospital, but never, not once, did she say anything about Clint being discharged from the facility. What she said was that they were struggling to keep Clint calm whenever he got ag-itated and said our family would need to figure out a better way of managing his care (implying while at the facility), especially his urge to get up out of his wheelchair.

I told her I was open to suggestions and reminded her of the suggestion from the facility director to purchase a bean bag where Clint would basically be sitting on the ground and unable to get up on his own to avoid falls. I also reminded her that I had already purchased a hockey helmet for him to wear to protect his head if or when he falls. The DON just said, "Well, we need to figure something out" and left it at that. I asked the night nurse what the expectation was for the ambulance to take him back to the hospital. She proceeded to tell me that it was not up to her, but I needed to understand she was not allowing Clint back into the facility. I reminded her that all his belongings, including the bed, were still in the facility. She basically told me I needed to work that out the following day when the day shift was on and gave the phone back to the EMT. I asked the EMT if he had ever experienced something like this, as I had no clue what to do. He told me he did not and asked me what I wanted him to do. I told him to take him back to the hospital. To say I was furious is an understatement. I was livid—and I was scared. "What am I supposed to do? What is the right decision here? Do I call law enforcement? Who can I call this time of night?"

I got home and began calling the director of nursing, but she did not answer. I called the director of the facility (as he gave me his personal cell number), still no answer. I called law enforcement and drove to a local restaurant to meet with an officer from the county that Clint was in to file a report. However, after speaking with them, I learned that there was nothing for them to do. The officer recommended I call the ombudsman for nursing homes.

Then, as I was driving home, it hit me.

While sitting at the hospital with Clint, I had picked up an AARP magazine with an article about underhanded strategies that nursing homes pull and the steps they take to kick out their "problem" residents. One strategy is to send them to the ER and arbitrarily discharge them from the facility without having to notify the family. Their intent is to send the resident in for "evaluation" with the hopes of the doctor admitting them. Once admitted, the facility has the flexibility to deny their reentry into the facility, ultimately discharging them without having to inform the family. This tactic is called "resident dumping." The article was written in April 2021, so it was a fresh article. You can read it here: https://www.aarp.org/caregiving/financial-legal/info-2021/nursing-home-dumping-lawsuit.html

I am just now rereading that article and just realized that AARP provided counsel to that resident's family to help sue the facility that was found in the wrong. I wasn't thinking clearly that evening, a Friday at midnight, as I was talking to the night nurse a second time to convince her she was wrong and had bad information and she needed to let my brother back into his room. The doctor did not admit him, because he was not exhibiting any unruly behavior to even warrant an evaluation, much less admission to the hospital. The facility sent Clint to the ER under the expectation that he would not be returning, ever. It was after midnight when I finally received a call from the night nurse that she spoke with the ER doctor and had him sign a report or documentation that Clint was being returned.

The EMTs had Clint in the back of their ambulance for over three hours, driving between the hospital and the assisted living facility. The night nurse then *commanded* the following from me: "I'm going to let your brother back into the facility, but this is what you need to understand. YOU are now responsible for his care." Still in shock from it all, this still threw me, so I asked, "What do you mean I am responsible for his care? He is in your facility. Are you telling me you will not tend to him—take him to the bathroom, feed him, bathe him? What does that mean?" She stated that they would not be moving him to join the rest of the residents and that he would remain in his bed. If we, the family, wanted him moved, we, the family, would need to come take care of it. I kid you not, I wanted so badly to throat-punch this woman! I demanded to speak with the director of nursing imme- diately, but that never happened.

Is this how professional medical personnel handle conflict? Through avoidance? Through sleight-of-hand tactics? Through threats and barring medical care and services? "Ya' damn skippy my brother will be out of that facility just as soon as I make the necessary preparations to move him back in with me!" I may be a Christian and a professional, but don't be surprised when you play games like this—I WILL take all necessary steps to bring this to light and do whatever is necessary to protect those for whom I am advocating!

My sister and I were at the facility the following morning at 10:30 a.m. They were true to their word; Clint was still in bed. I asked if anyone had given him breakfast, and they said, "No, he's been sleeping." Apparently, the night nurse gave him another extra dose of Seroquel to make sure he stayed asleep. Renée and I woke him up, changed his diaper and clothes, sat him up in bed, and fed him breakfast. I called the director of the facility. He acted like he knew NOTHING (which I'm sure was a lie!). I also called the ombudsman, who serves as an advocate for the families and the residents. She was just as appalled as we were at all that had happened. The result, however, was the night nurse was supposedly given a written reprimand. Nothing happened to the director of nursing.

I gave my 30 days' notice, and the director of the facility assured me that my family would not have to take care of him daily, that he would make sure the staff returned him to his normal routine. Of course, I did NOT take him at his word, and I would pop in unannounced as often as I could. And let's not forget his guardian angel, who watched over him during her shift, unbeknownst to anyone else. When she first introduced herself to Clint, letting him know she was watching over him, he struggled but got the words out to her and said, "I'm in hell. Thank you." That person is no longer working there because of the abuse she witnessed at that facility.

I also filed a complaint with the Florida Agency for Health Care Administration. It took them nearly six months to acknowledge the complaint, and that was only because I kept calling and inquiring about it. When they finally assigned someone to the case to investigate, how they investigated no longer applied. They can't tell the facility who they are looking for or what resident they are investigating. They must make it "random" by asking to review records of patients that have the same diagnosis or other similarities as Clint. That wasn't the case by the time the investigator got there, so it became a moot point. All at the sacrifice of Clint's well-being. The picture of Mom and Clint on the dedication page was taken the day Clint came home from that facility. Both Mom and Clint were so very happy to be together again. That sentiment would continue with their passing, which I will share later.

In case you are curious about the name and location of this facility, know that it really doesn't matter. What you need to understand and realize is that the experience my family had represents a systemic problem within nursing homes throughout the world. Placing a target on one bad facility would be irresponsible and a waste of time. I know there are facilities that are willing to put forth the extra effort to ensure their staff receive the proper and current training so that their residents are given the best care possible. They also ensure the "right" people are hired—meaning, people who have the patience and compassion, or the willingness to learn to properly care for those with dementia, instead of rashly hiring a warm body to meet the staff-to-resident ratio. And the leadership in place leads by example, showing compassion to their staff and ensuring their needs are met, as well. These are the facilities that deserve a target—a spotlight of "what RIGHT looks like."

Next, the powers that be need to pay attention to these good facilities—be it the entities that govern these facilities or the elected officials who influence the laws that are introduced to protect seniors living in these facilities and their families. Use these good facilities to establish the standard. Then create inspection guidelines based on these standards. Develop inspection teams to conduct random, unscheduled visits. And, yes, I realize the additional challenges of hiring to fill these additional roles. May I recommend reaching out to the veteran community? Veterans with a medical and/or especially an Inspector General background already have the training and understanding of this process. Veterans know what "right" looks like and they know how to conduct inspections. Veterans are also compassionate when it comes to working with families. They most definitely have experience in that department.

Within the first few days of Clint being home, I got COVID from one of the in-home healthcare workers. Charles and I had been on good terms, and he offered to come to help me take care of Clint and Mom. Having COVID, all in-home healthcare providers were not allowed to come into the home until we tested negative. Charles assured me he had already had COVID and was vaccinated. After he got COVID the second time, he chose to get the monoclonal antibodies and strongly urged me to do the same for all three of us, so I did. I also accepted Charles's offer to help me with Clint, as I was physically drained, and Clint was too much for Mom to care for. I lived five hours away, and Charles packed up and drove that evening. He worked remotely, and I had a home office for him to use, so within five hours, Charles was knocking on my door. Within three days of getting the monoclonal antibodies, I began feeling better and getting my strength back. Also, almost immediately, I saw a 180-degree change in Charles [from when we were married] soon after he arrived. His whole demeanor was softer, calmer, and he exuded a compassion I had not seen before. Only God knew the shift that was about to take place.

End of Chapter Takeaways

I offer a few key takeaways from this chapter. One is about the journey to becoming an advocate for your loved one. It involves first understanding what is happening to them and understanding all you can about the disease. Trust your instincts by digging deep into all you've learned in your own personal life that you can draw upon and use to help you in this moment. Ask yourself what experiences you have had and how they can best serve you and your loved one at this time.

Another key takeaway is patience and presence. It's important to be fully focused on the person you are caring for so that you can witness or catch their new or different behaviors that give you clues to something being out of the ordinary. With the busyness of today's society, or in my case while I was in the Army, I needed to remove myself from that environment and enter Clint's environment and be fully present to recognize things that neither Clint could share, nor the doctors could possibly know.

And if you've never been big on taking notes, know that you will need notes when you meet with doctors, nurses, facility di rectors, and even home health providers. I took a lot of notes. You'll need to write down the day and time a certain event happens, what precedes it, the effects of medicines, changes in behavior, even the difference in what medical personnel tell you and the intuitions they give. You'll find it all important.

It is imperative that you have an open line of communication with the staff of any institution to which your loved one is visiting, such as an emergency room. If the staff and the EMT personnel don't understand the world of dementia, they have no idea how to read the signs and symptoms and won't bother looking for a road map. *You* must give them that road map!

Stick to a routine as much as possible. You may not be able to predict someone's behavior, but you can control their medication by writing down all their medications and the amount and frequency they are to be given. That is a routine for you. Try to help them start and end their day around the same time and get to know their favorite foods. You can plan their meals around their favorite dishes to continue to give them a sense of familiarity. These are all efforts in developing a routine for them and you.

Also, don't be afraid to do a little research; ask questions, especially when you don't understand something. Whether that is medical personnel or government agency staff, when your loved one can no longer speak on their own behalf, you must be ready to find the courage to speak for them. If you have done your research, then you are better able to speak intelligently and defend your position on a matter. It may not mean you will always win an argument, but it will at least get you closer to a solution by creating dialogue with decision-makers. Doing nothing—saying nothing—does no one, especially your loved one, any good.

My final takeaway (I realize this was a lengthy chapter): remember your loved one is still inside. See them through the lens of knowing they are trying their best to communicate with you. Pay attention to their body language, as well as what they are saying. If you keep searching for "them," you will find them, and oh how it will warm your heart!

CHAPTER TWO
LIFE IS A JOURNEY

Life can only be understood backwards; but it must be lived forwards.
Life is not a problem to be solved, but a reality to be experienced.
(Søren Kierkegaard)

The first time I heard that quote, I was watching Pastor Dharius Daniels on YouTube. I had been caring for Clint for about four months. I immediately considered my life and all I had been through and experienced. I also considered Clint's life, with all his accomplishments and experiences, and the life he was now being forced to live. And then, of course, Mom's life. Had she ever pondered why her life turned out the way it did? Becoming a single mother of four children; a one-night stand that would produce a fifth child, then a personally proclaimed adoption of a sixth child? She nearly lost her second-oldest son at age 16 in a car crash because he had been drinking, killing another person in the vehicle, and sending his best friend through the windshield, cutting his skull within 1/16 inch of his brain. She then dealt with drive-by shootings because her young-est son didn't have a father figure around and sought guidance and significance from the neighborhood gangs, and their trou-bles found their way onto her doorstep.

The siblings rallied together and "volun-told" her to move to another state, out in the country where there would be peace and quiet, and family nearby to help when needed. She then cared for her own mother till she died, cared for her daughter-in-law till she died, then took her oldest son in to care for him until the can-cer told her "No more." What does life mean when faced with so many hardships? I never asked her prior to her moving in, and she never shared her deepest emotions, even after moving in with me. Not that I didn't try to break through her shell. I tried to get her to open up every day she lived with me. But there were 80 years' worth of layers to break through; it wasn't going to crack in only three years.

I have been on a journey of my own these last few years, seeking answers to questions such as that, to asking what "truth" is and what the purpose of life on Earth is. It has taken me down some interesting paths that have ventured out beyond the Bible and questioning everything I was raised on. I was in this mindset when Charles came to help me with Clint. But that wasn't the topic of discussion at that moment. He was there to help me with Clint and help he did. I was so very grateful for his newfound patience and compassion. I found my eyes and my heart seeing and feeling the man I fell in love with 23 years prior. I don't think it took 24 hours to find us falling into this natural rhythm of simply moving throughout the day —from cleaning, to cooking, to taking care of honey-dos, even though I didn't ask. I imagine it would've been amazing to watch the two of us do this life dance together, but it was much more amazing to feel it and experience it. We were beginning to fall back in love again. We had many tough conversations about "what happened" and "why the divorce." He ended up staying about a month, and by the second month, he proposed to me again, and I said "Yes!" We remarried a few months later but spent the first year having intentional and meaningful conversations to rebuild trust and establish the direction of our relationship. And we did reach out to our kids to get their permission to remarry! We talked to them individually, and hilariously enough they both said the same thing: "Just agree now that if it doesn't work, don't call us—let it go and move on!" We laughed. We agreed and couldn't be happier. Life truly is a journey.

Windows of Time
For the longest time, prior to Clint's diagnosis, my relationship with Clint was amiable. There were six years between us, and aside from having chores to do around the house or going to our dads in the summers, he had his circle of friends, and I had mine. But I respected him because he was so smart, he went into the military, and he got to see new places outside of Jacksonville. "He got away!" and I thought it was a good plan.

When Clint was reassigned from Japan to Maryland, he got married soon after arriving. He was still living there when I graduated high school. I knew Clint and his wife would be coming down for the holidays, so I asked if I could live with them until I found a job and could get my own place. I knew there wasn't much to offer me if I stayed in Jacksonville. I wanted a better life for myself too.

I ran in a variety of circles in high school. Some of those circles came from families in the middle class, some above, and some below. As far as I knew, my family was below middle class. Crime was increasing in my neighborhood, and I knew many teenage girls who were pregnant by age 16 and struggling financially and relationally. I didn't quite know what "right" looked like at age 18, but I was certain there was something better waiting for me away from Westside. I had recently turned 18 when Clint and his wife came home for Christmas. I loaded up my car and followed him home just before the New Year.

I come from a family of hard workers—and I learned that lesson well. Since our parents were divorced, during the summers we would stay with our dad in Georgia. We each had our turn, but when we were old enough, we worked in the tobacco fields. It gave us spending money, and Daddy knew it would instill discipline and a strong work ethic in us. I began working at age 13, tying the tobacco to sticks as it was pulled off the stalks and then pulling it off the sticks once it dried in the barn. I wasn't old enough to sit in the seats and pull the leaves from the stalks. I'm sure I hated working in the fields and getting the tar on my fingers at the time, but in hindsight, it was some of the best memories. The farm owner's wife would prepare lunch, and there would be about 10–15 of us sitting at a long table eating some of the best Southern cooking: homemade biscuits, fried chicken, and sweet tea. We'd sit on the grass during a break and eat fresh watermelon from their garden. Then some of the guys who were pulling tobacco leaves would find their rhythm, singing songs or a cadence to make the work seem lighter and go faster.

Once I moved in with Clint and his wife, I worked during the day as a customer service representative for a food service company and as a waitress at night. Clint and I had an agreement that I would pay the extra amount on their light and water bill and a minimal amount per month for rent. I lived with them for about six months and saved enough money to get my own apartment, but I stayed out of their way as much as possible to not interrupt their routine. Unfortunately, no matter how hard I tried and thought I was giving them space, my sister-in-law always felt burdened by my presence, and I could feel the tension and the conflict in my brother's soul. I was his baby sister, but she was his wife, and a spouse always takes precedence. I was hurt by some of the accusations she made toward me and worked more hours to stay out of their hair and to save more money, faster. After six months, I found my own apartment.

I didn't have any furniture, but I bought an air mattress, a pot, a pan, a few dishes, and a couple of towels and washcloths. I was doing pretty well at adulting for an 18-year-old, but I really didn't have a plan, and I had no idea what my future would hold.

After I moved out, Clint suggested I move back home to Mom's in Florida, where I would be around people I knew and be closer to people who could help me if I needed it. Ultimately, he was saying "he" couldn't or wouldn't be there to help me when I needed it. To me, moving home would be a "failure" in my mind—something I refused to accept—so I worked that much harder to continue living on my own.

I soon became involved in a relationship with a guy from work and followed him to Miami, where his brother lived. I lived in Miami for about 18 months (the relationship didn't last) then moved back to the area where Clint lived but slept on a friend's couch temporarily. I got my old waitress job back but needed a more permanent solution to "three hots and a cot" (food and a place to sleep) and a job that would provide for me.

My favorite cousin was in the Army National Guard, and she suggested joining the Army full-time. I had considered joining the Air Force like Clint when I graduated high school, but I wanted to go into computers, and they didn't have any of those jobs available. I never considered it again until my cousin suggested joining the Army—with my family background, it seemed natural. So, I walked into a recruiter's office and asked, "Where do I sign and how soon can I leave?" I shipped off to basic training about three weeks later, leaving my belongings at Clint's house.

After I completed my initial training, I found myself assigned just north of where Clint lived. Funny, actually; I was 20 years old when I joined the military, and they ask you to list three places you would like to be assigned—a wish list, if you will. I was so ready to just "get out of Dodge" I wrote "Germany. Germany. Germany" for all three options of where I would like to go. Most 18-year-olds who join the military typically list their hometown or places close enough on their wish list but usually get shipped overseas. I thought I had a much better chance of going overseas if I told them that's where I "wanted" to go. But, no! I ended up being stationed within 50 miles of where I entered the military! In hindsight, God knew what would be happening 30 years later. *His* steps were being laid out.

I tried reaching out to Clint a few times to chat, but he was distant. So, one day I showed up on his doorstep to find out what was going on. He had kept my hope chest with some of my personal things for me when I moved. The Gulf War had just started, and I was confused as to why he was avoiding me. He then shared with me that his wife accused me of stealing towels when I moved out. Even though I didn't take them, he didn't let me in the house because of her missing towels. I was done trying to convince him that I was innocent. Having the "matter-of-fact" personality that I have, I was done asking for permission to get my own belongings. I told him that I was backing my car up to his garage and loading my things. I reminded him that we were both in the military and that a war just started, and either of us could go downrange—military term for being close to the war front—and never return. So, I asked, "Are you sure this is how you want to leave our relationship?" He said, "Of course not... I don't know what to do." I hugged and kissed him goodbye. The only time we saw each other after that was during family gatherings, which were few and far between. But slowly, we rebuilt that missing connection, starting around the time he retired.

Clint began and ended his military career in Japan. He bought a Harley, and he talked about riding through the mountains of Japan and the beauty he saw. He had an opportunity to get promoted one more time to the highest enlisted rank of E-9. But he had had enough and was ready to be free from the military and do his own thing. He always talked about wanting to retire in Georgia, where our father is from and where we spent a lot of our time as kids during the summers. Our other brother, Marcus, lived there with his wife. The lifestyle is at a much slower pace than Washington, DC, or Jacksonville, Florida, where we grew up. Clint and Marcus loved working on Clint's motorcycle and old cars together, so retirement to Georgia made sense to him.

Through all this, Clint's pride and joy were his girls: a daughter he didn't know for 18 years and two granddaughters he helped welcome into this world. His daughter lived in Florida, so he bought a house and retired there to be closer. There is a remarkably interesting story about Clint's daughter, Amy, that I will share a little later, in her own words.

All our siblings attended the same high school, and in 2010 the reunion committee, of which Clint was on, decided to do an "All-Eighties" reunion for everyone who graduated between 1980 and 1989. This captured the four of us, except for our oldest sister Renée. She graduated in 1978 but knew everyone, so she came too. We have two other siblings I haven't discussed much about. When I was 15 years old, my mom, at age 43, learned that some uncomfortable indigestion she was having was actually a baby! She was the talk of the maternity ward at the hospital in 1983: a 44-year-old gave birth to a healthy baby boy! I got to name him Corey. He was born one week after her birthday. The sixth sibling is one of my closest childhood friends, Karla. When I was in the seventh grade (about 12 years old), her family moved out of the school district, and she moved in with me to stay at the same school. Mom became her "in loco parentis." Karla has been considered our adopted sister ever since. But neither Karla nor Corey attended our All-Eighties class reunion—only the four of us.

We had a great family and high school reunion that year. Clint was the emcee and looked so dapper in his tuxedo. Just another wonderful experience for him, and a memory for us. And it was during this weekend that Clint and I reconnected more. He enjoyed being the center of attention, and he was a very handsome man with a beautiful smile. I'm so grateful for the pictures we took that year, not only of the reunion but our time together as a family. To see Clint's smile and hear his laughter would brighten anyone's day. He was happy, and it showed.

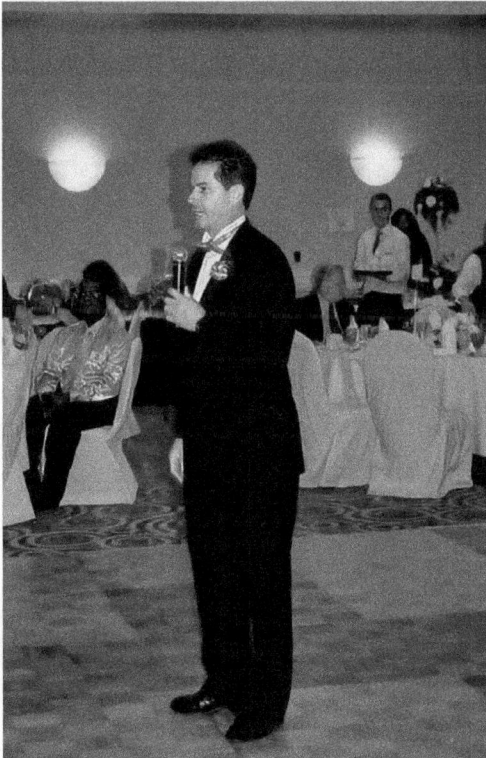

Clint in full dress as the Emcee for our High School Reunion, 2010

In addition to the high school reunion, the four of us also did a Bible study together on a DVD series called The Truth Project. Excellent study! We each had our questions, doubts, as well as strengths about faith, God, Christ, and the Bible. However, from the privacy of our own home, we intimately shared in conversation via phone conferences and email, and participated as a family where we had never done anything like that "together" before. It was refreshing and a moment of bonding that brought us closer than we ever had.

I look back at those reunion pictures now and think about where each of us were living, where we were in our careers, or our family life and plans for the future. None of us had any inclination about what was waiting for each of us just five years in the future or how drastic our lives would change (within our control) or be changed (outside of our control). I know Clint did not. He was living his best life by developing his relationship with God, watching his granddaughters grow up, working at a local hospital, and going on bike rallies with his Harley.

God has always been a part of our lives, in some way, shape, or form, and we believe in Jeremiah 29:11: "For I know the plans I have for you," declares the Lord, "plans to prosper you and not to harm you, plans to give you hope and a future." As believers in Christ, we stand on the promises of God. Yet still, things happen that cause us to ask, "Why?" if not "Why me?" or "Why now?"

What are you supposed to do when your reality becomes so vastly different from the reality you once knew or different from everyone around you? What happens when there is a shift in your path and you are no longer moving forward, but backward?

Life truly is a journey. Søren Kierkegaard said it best, *"Life can only be understood backwards; but it must be lived forwards. Life is not a problem to be solved, but a reality to be experienced."* Clint experienced life and had some amazing rewards along the way, from his success in the military and experiencing another country's culture, cuisine, and countryside, to his daughter and granddaughters. Even his marriage had great memories. I believe Clint lived "forward" until life began slowing down and he didn't understand why or what was happening.

I realize we all have unfulfilled dreams. We do not think about it or really internalize it until the loss begins around us. Death makes you think about what you forgot to do in life, leading to regrets or igniting dreams that can still happen.

Forever Friendships
Clint had many, many friends, but two people who wanted to share some of their greatest memories were his girlfriend, Kathy, and one of his best friends from the Air Force, Jim. Here are their stories.

Meet Kathy:
Glad I Got to Know You

Death ends a life, not a relationship. All the love you created is still there. All the memories are still there. You live on—in the hearts of everyone you have touched and nurtured while you were here.
~ Morrie Schwartz

December 23, 2023

My dearest Clint,

As my family prepares for Christmas 2023, I recall our first Christmas with you in 2011. I can picture you jingling bells in the middle of the night so that Noah and Gabe might believe that Santa and his reindeer had landed on our roof. Although you left our neighborhood almost seven years ago and our earthly world eight months ago, you continue to occupy a special place in our hearts and minds. As Morrie Schwartz reminds us, "Death ends a life, not a relationship." We can no longer see your smile or hear your laughter, but we still feel your eternal love and cherish the memories that we made with you. Our spiritual relationship with you will endure long after your time in this world. Beloved friend and father figure, you live on in our daily thoughts, words, and deeds.

Shortly after your death, your sister Julie invited me to share reflections about you in a book that she is writing to honor your life and legacy. As I compose this letter, I am looking at a bright pink satchel filled with cards, pictures, and other mementos from you. Years ago, I organized these keepsakes chronologically, from your first card in July 2011 to your last one in February 2017.

I treasure each handwritten note from you. One that seems especially fitting for this occasion reads, "Life's a journey . . . glad we're in it together!" I remain grateful for the journey, however fleeting, that the boys and I shared with you.

Early on our journey, I noticed that you sometimes struggled to remember a name or to find your keys. As your condition progressed, you asked me to sit down with you and record some of your favorite sayings, which I called "Clint-isms." You were concerned that you would not be able to remember those sayings in the future and you wanted me to help you preserve them for your loved ones. Regrettably, I never made the time to have that conversation with you. I took our moments together for granted, and before long, you moved to Douglas, Georgia, to live with your mom.

I yearn to have one more conversation with you while we sip on your incomparably delicious coffee (you were a world-class barista!). I am certain that you would help me to complete the list of Clint-isms more accurately, and of course, you would add your clever wit and charming humor to the experience. I humbly ask that you accept the belated list of your favorite sayings and my explanations of them:

Clint's Favorite Sayings and Kathy's Explanations

Clint's Saying	Kathy's Explanation
Glad you got to see me.	Clint loved making other people smile and laugh. This saying was his hallmark tongue-in-cheek way of saying "goodbye" or "see you later."

Stop and smell the roses.	Clint believed in taking time to enjoy nature. He encouraged others to take a picture of a beautiful sunset or a blooming tree whenever possible.
Walk slowly and confidently.	Trained in the Air Force to walk with poise, Clint wanted others to do the same. He felt that walking too quickly revealed fear and anxiety that could draw negative attention, particularly for women.
ちょっと待って	These characters are Japanese for "wait a second," pronounced "chottomatte." Clint often told his two German shepherds, Garren and Tanzer, to wait a second in Japanese. Clint occasionally used this expression when asking Noah and Gabe to wait for a meal, a game of ball, or a trip to the movies. Clint learned this expression when he was stationed as an airman in Japan. There was a second part to the expression, but unfortunately, I could not recall it.
Check your six.	Clint learned this expression in the Air Force. He encouraged others to be aware of their surroundings, especially from behind. He offered this advice in both a literal and figurative sense.
Keep your head on a swivel.	Clint encouraged his family and friends to look frequently to the left and right as well as to the rear when driving. He compared the head and eye movements of effective drivers to being on a swivel.
Good looks good.	Clint believed that a woman could be beautiful at any age, not just when young. In his eyes, facial lines and gray hair did not detract from a woman's beauty.
You're Mom.	Clint believed in empowering moms, especially single moms of boys, with the

	knowledge that they already have all the authority that they need to command their children's respect and raise them to be good men.
Everyone needs a witness to their life.	Clint loved the 2004 movie Shall We Dance? A theme from this movie that resonated with him is that we all need someone who truly sees us . . . who loves us . . . and who shares life with us.
You blink and it goes by just like that.	Clint often commented on how quickly life goes by. As he entered his fifties, he could hardly believe how much time had passed in his own life.
God is good all the time . . . and all the time God is good.	Clint and I took Noah and Gabe to see the movie God's Not Dead around 2014. He learned this expression from the movie, and he often quoted it. In February 2013, when Clint was 50, he gave his life to Christ and became a born-again Christian. To this day, Clint's faith in God is the purest and deepest that I have ever witnessed.
I'm still here.	When Clint struggled to remember details and to speak, he often said, "I'm still here" as a way of letting others know that he was able to understand and communicate even if he was "stammering," as he referred to his speech difficulties.
I know where I'm going.	Around 2016, when Clint learned that he had frontal-temporal lobe dementia, he expressed fear that he might die young, perhaps in his sixties. When he said, "I know where I'm going," he was referring to Heaven. He believed that God had a plan for his life and that he was Heaven-bound after his time on Earth.

I hope that I did justice to this long-delayed exercise in re-calling your favorite expressions, and I also hope that these sayings help others as much as they have the boys and me.

Quick-witted, you always had the right word at the right time. In your first card to me, you wrote, "Glad we finally met." I am grateful that I got to meet you and know you—to witness you. You remain one of the most influential people in my life and my boys' lives. Shortly after we met, you penned the words "Looking forward to our journey!" on a greeting card that featured a frog aboard a boat made of newspaper. Because of you, I know where I'm going on my life journey, and I am looking forward to joining you when I get there.

With love always,

Kathy

P.S. Almost every card that you gave me included your signature character—a hand-drawn figure with stalks of spikey hair, elfin ears, and wonder-filled eyes. I sent Julie a copy of the character so that she could include it in your memory book. I once asked you about the meaning of the figure, and true to your artistic nature, you didn't answer me directly. Instead, you softly smiled and said that you had been drawing it for years. I have come to believe that the character represented you—a one-of-a-kind soul who may have sometimes felt as if he were on the outside looking into a world to which he did not entirely belong. To me, your long-suffering and early departure from this life reveal that you were meant for a much greater world—for Heaven, where you have become one of God's angels.

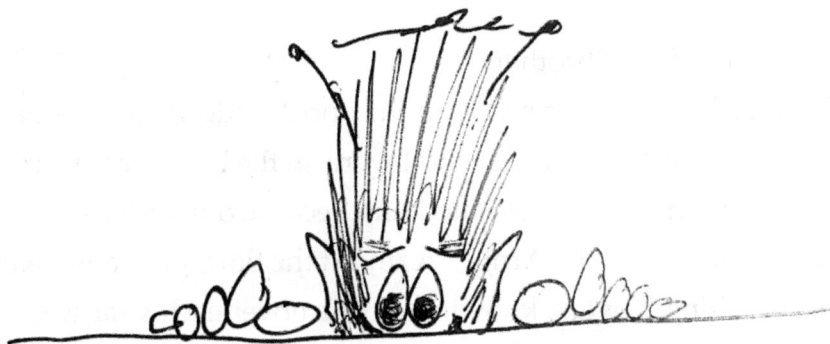

Clint's signature drawing

Thank you, Kathy. When I first began reading your memories, the phrase you wrote about "life being a journey," I couldn't help but smile and tear up. It was the title for this chapter, and I immediately heard the whisper, "You are right where you are supposed to be."

Out of curiosity, I researched what the second part of the Japanese phrase of Chotto Matte was, and the word is Kuda Sai, meaning "please," as found on the Quora website, which states the following:

What does "Chatto matte" mean and how is it used? It's short for "Chatto matte kudasai" and means "please wait a bit." The "kudasai" is the "please," so you don't leave it off lightly, even though nothing else could sensibly follow a -te form in that context. Sep. 18, 2015

Clint taught politeness. He loved his experiences in Japan and their culture, and politeness is part of their culture.

Meet Jim

In memory of my "brother"

I met Clint playing soccer in the Fort Meade soccer league in the summer of 1982. John C. and I were on the USAF team. I can't remember which team recruited him because our roster was full. I believe he was on the Army's team. At the time, John and I were still recruiting players, knowing our turnover each year was between a third to half the team. We watched Clint play. He was their best player, maybe the only one who truly had foot skills.

So, John and I did what we knew best: harass the guy we wanted, to test his character. We practically mauled Clint on the field. I recall both John and I tackling him, and he popped up with a surprised look, red-faced, while John and I were smiling. "We want you to come play for us, Clint." When the game ended, we hung around and put away a lot of beers and made it official.

The three of us bonded and drew several more elite players to our team. Our team dominated the league, winning the championship five years straight from '82 to '86. We also put together a team in one of the toughest leagues in the state, Division I, Howard County outdoor league. We eventually won it all there too. During that time, we played two to three outdoor soccer games a week. When the weather changed, we played two to three indoor soccer games a week in several leagues where we dominated: in Columbia, MD, at the ice rink; in downtown Baltimore at Fells Point; at an indoor facility in Parkville; and one in Sykesville. We even had semi-pro players joining our indoor team, and we were approached by a coach from the Polish national team who wanted to coach us, but we decided we liked what we had with the three of us managing our teams.

Clint and I played strikers, John was our stopper/midfield shutdown defender. Our goalies came and went, so Clint and I alternated, until we picked up Scott W. for our outdoor leagues only. And to be honest, I trusted Clint as a goalie more than myself. I'd had a couple ugly injuries, and I would only play goalie if none of our others showed.

We were young, newly married, and really only knew our coworkers and teammates. We hung out and cooked out with Clint and his wife, Patti; John and Jill (girlfriend at the time); me and Carol (my wife) through the mid-'80s until I left the service. We put away a lot of beers, watched too many movies, and laughed our asses off countless numbers of times. We reconnected a year later when I came back as a civilian and Clint was assigned to Andrews AFB. John went overseas. At that time, it became just Clint and Patti, their dogs Shorty and Shena, about a dozen ferrets, and some cats. We had dogs as well. It was easier for us to go hang at their townhome in Columbia, which we did most weekends. The cookouts, games we played, Clint's Coors Light fetish—I could never get him to drink Guinness with me and John, LOL. Our military soccer highlight was when the three of us in the USAF got to play the Army in an exhibition game before a Baltimore Blast game. We beat and shut out the Army. Clint was our goalie. Nothing got by him. I managed to score a goal. John was stellar on defense and assists.

Before John left, after we won our final Fort Meade championship together, our outdoor goalie Scott threw a monster party at his house and property in Jessup. It ran for two days straight. I have pics somewhere. Clint and I drove around the property, picking up passed-out teammates in the fields. We found one chained to a tree with no pants. We're not sure how it happened, but it took us forever to get him off that tree because we couldn't stop laughing. Clint, Patti, her sister Ann, Carol, and I left the party to go see Heart at Merriweather Post Pavilion. Someone got lawn seats, and we had a blast there for hours. When we returned, we had to go look for the people we rescued earlier. One had managed to go upstairs and climb into a laundry basket and got stuck.

I never cried so hard from laughing. We took turns hosing them off outside. It took another day to remove and clean that poor house. I could always count on Clint to help whenever we needed, and vice versa. Clint and I both took up refereeing as well as playing. It opened doors and opportunities for both of us in Maryland. I ended up taking a transfer to western NC two years later, about the time John returned. Clint kept up with John and ran the leagues I was running with them.

In 1991, my wife had our first child. It was a C-section, and my son was difficult to say the least. We found out later that he was on the spectrum for autism, but highly functioning. He still lives with us and works for the NHL. Clint and Patti showed up the day after his birth. They were at a timeshare 30 minutes away. They invited us out, but we couldn't go. I felt bad at the time, as we lost touch while out there for five years. It was a tough time. We moved back to Maryland after our daughter was born and reconnected in the '90s. Clint played on my Sykesville indoor team for a while. I saw Clint when we played, but we never reconnected as a couple. Having two small kids changes your perspective and outlook. My focus was on them, getting a good education and then hopefully off to college. That plan didn't work out until much later. I saw more of John than I did of Clint, but I think he may have moved to Jacksonville in the 2000s.

We moved to Virginia in 2012 as I took another transfer. I began visiting my FLA snow birding parents for a week during the winters. I think I found Clint in 2013 or 2014 and promised to come see him on my next trip down. We met up at a Hooters in Jacksonville in 2015. We spent several hours catching up there, but I had a hard time focusing on him, LOL. It was great catching up; it was like seeing my brother. I was actually closer to Clint and John than my older brother. What has been great about John and Clint is that we would pick up where we left off and not miss a beat. No drama, just friends having a great time. I always wished that he could have stayed up in Maryland with us.

When John called me to let me know Clint was suffering from dementia and had moved back to Georgia, I was shocked. John wanted to come down once he came back from the UAE, but I was dealing with some medical issues. I was awestruck to find out that Clint had a brother and sister. I never knew.

John and I both know each other's parents and siblings. I'm not sure why Clint never shared that. I knew something had happened between him and Patti, as he told me some of it, but I didn't pry or push him to tell me more. I was trying to be respectful of what he wanted me to know. I guess the trauma of it all affects everyone differently. As I reflect on our friendship, it sticks with me some, because it's the most current memory I have of Clint, but I am choosing to remember him in those carefree days when he would break into a huge smile if he saw me or John. He was a huge part of my twenties and thirties, and I'm beyond grateful to have known him and call him my "brother from another mother." I love you, Clint. I always will. See you when my time is called. ♥

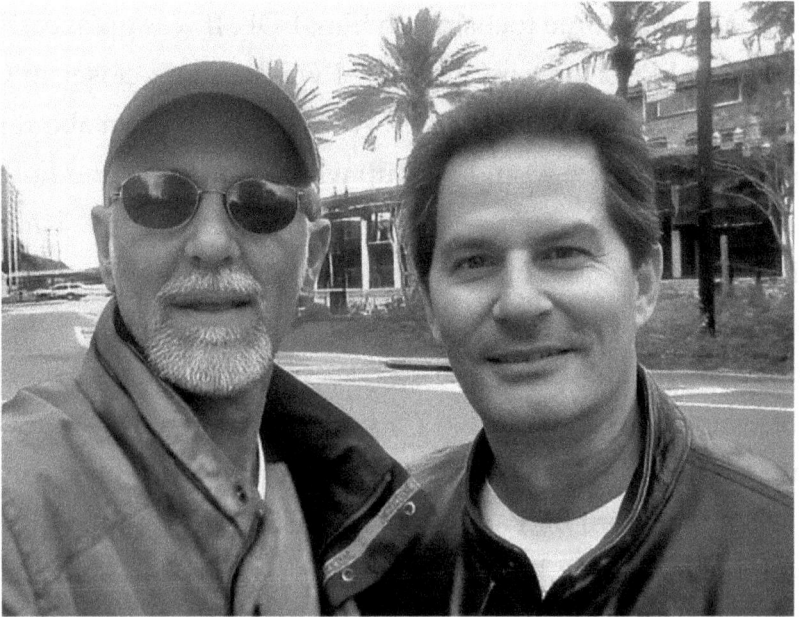

Jim and Clint

Oh, my goodness! Thank you, Jim, for those memories. Reading them allowed me to peek into another side of Clint I did not get to see or know. I laughed and cried right along with you. Clint was always my "intelligent, older brother with a very important job in the Air Force." As you mentioned above, when life hits you and you begin having kids of your own, your focus shifts. We will never know why Clint never shared with you how many siblings he had or any other personal information about his family. I can speculate and suggest that maybe because he knew we would never meet, so it was inconsequential, or maybe his life with the military and his wife were sacred and he chose to keep it separate from his family. What I can say is Clint loved life, and he chose to live it on his terms—until he couldn't. Thank you for being his best friend and giving him memories to hold on to in his darkest moments.

Clint's Pride and Joy

Talk about a beautiful story. First, Clint was not only known for his brains, percussion, and dancing skills, but he was also a handsome young man! Many people have that one love they met in high school; "true love" is what they call it. Clint found that someone when he was a junior, but for whatever reason, it didn't work out—she ended up moving away, and Clint moved on. After graduating high school, he joined the military and married three years later. But one day, 18 years after graduating, Clint received a phone call where his past met him in his future. Her name was Amy Christine, and she was a daughter he never knew he had. Here is Amy's account and a few memories she shared of the man in a picture that her mom gave her when she was little, telling her, "This is Clint; he is your dad."

Amy's story

The first memory I have of him is when I met him for the first time. I was living in Pensacola at the time, and he flew me up to Maryland to meet him. I was 18. I had searched my whole life for my biological father. My mom had always told me his name, and I had an old picture of him I used to look at all the time. It was from the '70s; he was standing with a group of people and was wearing those knee-high tube socks, lol. I was very nervous but excited at the same time. When I got off the plane, he was standing there with a dozen yellow roses (my favorite, by the way), and we embraced and stayed there holding each other for a long time. I remember many details from that trip as I was thinking of him. As we got in his red Jeep Cherokee to head to his house, I remember him wearing his sunglasses with the straps on them to hang around his neck, his watch on his arm, and I watched him drumming on the steering wheel to the beat of the music. I thought, 'My dad is so handsome and cool!' I met his 12 cats. I learned every one of their names and personalities. My favorite was Drac (Dracula) because he would always suck my neck. During that trip, we took walks down the path behind his house holding hands, went to Washington DC and saw all the sights. We held the White House between our hands in a picture and then saw the national fireworks from Andrews AFB. I remember some of them were smiley faces in the sky (I thought that was so cool). We went into Baltimore to a seafood restaurant on the water and he taught me how to crack and eat crab legs because I had never had them before. Now I'm a master at crab leg cracking. I learned that we both had the same favorite cereal, Lucky Charms, and we had the same feet, chin, and butt, lol. I didn't want to come home because I had so much fun and didn't want it to end. Patty (his wife at the time) made us shirts with our picture and the date of our first visit that I wore home on the plane. He gave me a little jewelry box with the dried-up yellow roses in the glass on the top of it to take home.

I remember at my wedding with the girl's dad—not too long after I first met him. He still lived in Maryland at the time. I think we had still only met for the first time. He was upset that he didn't walk me down the aisle; my stepdad did. So, when the pastor asked who gives this woman away and my stepdad said, "Her mother and I do," my dad stood up and firmly said, "I do," then sat down. I didn't realize until that moment that it was something he wanted, and I was just getting to know him, but it had always stuck in my head.

Very soon after that, he moved to Gautier, MS, which was about two hours away from Pensacola. We started taking turns driving to each other's houses on the weekends, and we would go to this place on the water to eat. I don't remember the name, but it was so cute, and you could drive your boat up and dock it and go eat. We used to take his boat out a lot and go there.

He was there, in the room, while I gave birth to my first daughter, Chasity, in Pensacola. He was so proud to be a grandpa, and he was so good with her. We spent Christmas together that year for the first time.

We moved to Jacksonville, and he went to Japan for a while. He would send me pictures of his motorcycle he bought and I'ete' (his cat), and I remember missing him a lot. But then when he came back, he moved to Jacksonville near me. He first had an apartment and then bought a house to be near us. It was across the street from the girls' elementary school so that he could pick them up sometimes.

He bought me my first bottle of wine and I hated it at first but learned to love it. We would have a glass of wine together when he came over.

We hung out every week, a couple times a week, either at each other's houses or we would go out to eat. Our favorite place was Whitey's fish camp in Middleburg. We would watch the manatees swimming around while we ate.

We would always put music on and dance. He was a really good dancer, and it was something we shared and loved doing together. We went out to clubs a few times and danced. (My husband didn't like that too much, lol) We would just laugh and joke and enjoy each other—making up for lost time.

When my ex-husband lost his job, we had to move to Texas. I didn't want to go, and I know that made him sad… It made me sad too. I came to visit as much as I could, but I did notice that his calls and messages started to become less and less, and he kept apologizing, saying he was not a very good dad. He always called me "daughter"—like "hi daughter" or "how are you doing, daughter," hahaha. I told him he was not a bad father at all. He said he would try to be better. Looking back, I think he was already having some neurological issues, and we had not realized it yet. Then the stuttering started, and you know the rest.

I knew when I got married to Mikael, he HAD to walk me down the aisle—no ifs, ands, or buts about it. I knew it was something he had always wanted to do. I was so proud to have him do that. I can't thank y'all enough. (Picture taken three years after diagnosis)

I miss our hour-long phone conversations. I miss our outings and our dinner parties. I miss his laugh, his jokes, and the little man he used to draw on all of the letters and cards he would give me. I miss him dancing. I just miss him and wish Mike would have gotten to know him before he got sick.

~"daughter," Amy

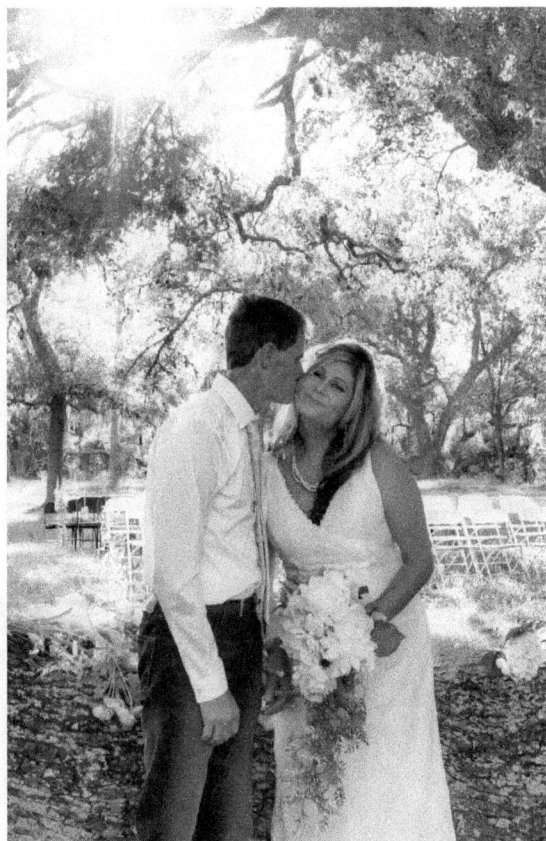

Clint & Amy, Father of the Bride Moment, 2019

End of Chapter Takeaways

All families have their challenges and struggles. But at the end of the day, family is family, and it is my belief that families have a devotion, if not obligation, to one another. What's even more important is that sometimes we forget that we are all human beings on this same journey called life. We make choices and decisions every day; some we are proud of, some we are not. We all make mistakes. Forgiveness is such a powerful action one can take to help our souls heal. It then allows us to see humanity in others— their weaknesses and need to feel loved. The key takeaway here is to forgive any past conflicts that may be keeping you from helping your family members in their time of need, especially with a debilitating disease.

No one "deserves" to die alone.

PART TWO

BALANCING LIFE'S CHALLENGES
AND LESSONS LEARNED

E very generation of elderly people has had their share of challenges. Today's challenges, however, seem to be getting harder and harder to overcome. Concerns about Social Security being stopped and having enough medical insurance to cover all that comes with aging are always top of mind. There is also the concern of developing the one disease that slowly takes your life away: Alzheimer's. When most people reach their retirement years, they dream of "fun in the sun" or travel or relaxing and enjoying the grandkids. "Best laid plans," as the saying goes, means life deals you a different hand, and my mom was dealt a doozie. Navigating life with a terminal disease, on a fixed income, caring for two disabled adults, and managing the finances of a third disabled adult sounds like some exaggerated Dad story. "When I was your age, I walked to school, uphill, in the snow, and for five miles—both ways...." Sad to say, Mom's story is by no means exaggerated. Although it is a sad situation, it is a story of grit and determination, and compassion.

Mom was born with a gift of servitude. She loved being a nurse and loved it when the neighborhood kids would come to her with their skinned knees. Until the age of fifteen, I was the baby of four. It is my belief that if you are a parent of more than one child, your first child helps you find your footing as a parent, but by the time you hit baby number four, you have routines down and can relax some.

There are eight years between my oldest sibling, Renée, and me, which meant that by the time she was about ten (if not earlier), she assumed the babysitter role a lot of the time.

I know we had other babysitters (I've heard some stories), but I don't remember them because I was too young. Mom worked the graveyard shift so she could sleep while we were in school and be home when we got home. I never got the full story about how Mom was able to do it, but she enrolled me in first grade at age five, skipping kindergarten and graduating at age 17. The only person I remember "being in charge" was Renée when Mom was not home. I've often wondered if Mom got permission from the school to allow me to start school in first grade because of her work schedule. Things were different in the early '70s.

Mom worked hard, as any single mother does. She depended on us kids to do what we were told and taught by doing the right thing—staying out of trouble so she could continue to work and put food on the table. She expected us to do our chores to help her around the house so she could focus on things we couldn't do, like having a job to make money and pay the light and water bill, buy groceries, and take us to the doctor's office when needed. Many kids today don't receive the same lessons I learned growing up. I was doing laundry in elementary school, ironing my own clothes, and working in tobacco fields at the age of 13.

By age 15, I began hosting at a local restaurant and serving as a waitress by age 16. I then worked two jobs soon after graduating high school. I taught my kids to do laundry by the time they were in the third or fourth grade. When our son went to college, he was doing his own laundry, and many of his friends were like, "Dude! How do you know how to wash clothes! Can you teach me?" My response to my son was "You're welcome." And to my mom, "Thank you!"

Renée and I have had a few conversations in the last year or so about our different experiences with our parents growing up. Renée recalls butting heads a lot with Mom growing up (the "first born" perspective), while I recall Mom's lack of attention (the "youngest" perspective). We spent our summers with our dad, and some of my most prominent memories are waking up early, working on the tobacco farms, eating boiled peanuts and fresh watermelon from the roadside stand. Then the not-so-good memories of Momma and Daddy quizzing us when we returned from the other's home about the other's actions. I recall around the age of nine telling both to "stop asking me questions!" Our dad was quite authoritarian. You didn't talk back to him about anything, and we were often afraid to speak our minds—until I found the courage to tell him and Mom what I felt.

Renée and I found it special when Daddy or Momma spent time with us. One memory I have from one of my stays with Daddy was him living in a log house with no hot water. The first night we stayed there, we all slept in the front room near the fireplace. We had eaten fried chicken that night and left the trash on the front porch. Raccoons (or something) woke us up in the middle of the night when something crashed on the front porch. We were in the middle of the woods, so the only light was the moonlight. Oftentimes Daddy would get up early to head off to work. He would ask me the night before if I wanted to get up and go to breakfast with him, but that meant waking up between 3:30 a.m. and 4:00 a.m. We would ride into town and go to this small mom-and-pop restaurant, sit at a diner-like bar, and have breakfast together. Just me and him. Then, since there was no hot water in the cabin, Daddy rigged up a makeshift shower in the backyard with a water hose and a shower head, then erected a round frame to secure a shower curtain. We couldn't take a shower until late afternoon to allow the water hose, lying in the sun, to heat up. You had about five minutes of hot water!

I am grateful for the lessons I learned from both my mom and my dad. They are what shaped my character and gave me the foundation and drive to be successful. However, after having Mom live with me for three years under my care, I realized I did not know my mom that well. I knew her as the mom I grew up with when I was a little girl —the kind of mom that preferred watching soap operas over reading me a book or discussing homework, much less, what to do with my future when I graduated high school. I wanted her to spend time with me. I now realize she did the best she could do at the time. She made me a prom dress; she also helped make some of my baton-twirling costumes and let me participate in sports. But I left home when I was eighteen and never went back except for the very occasional visit.

With Mom living with me, I wanted to get to know "Carol" better. I wanted to understand what she enjoyed, what made her smile, and what she ultimately wanted in life. The problem was she struggled to express her emotions. Simply asking her, "What would you like to do today?" didn't exactly evoke a simple response. The best I could do was try and put myself in her shoes and consider what her responses might be based on her current situation. She could no longer drive, she lived with her daughter hundreds of miles away from her home and land that was "hers" and the people that had become her closest friends and family. And let us not forget, she had stage four cancer in her spine and brain and was on a multitude of medications and vitamins, dealing with the aftereffects of chemo and radiation. And, as if that weren't enough, her oldest son was living with advanced stages of dementia. This became my new perspective as I strived to understand how to bring her peace and joy.

Momma enjoyed being able to go to the beach or sit by the pool after moving in with me in Florida. I tried to plan time for just the two of us and schedule manicures and pedicures. Just like her shiny and sparkly jewelry, her pink or red nails always had to have glitter in them so they could be sparkly too! I also took her to get a massage a few times. Boy, she loved that!

We got all her medical records transferred to Moffitt Cancer Center in Tampa, Florida. They did a wonderful job of managing the cancer tumors in her brain and spine. The cancer was only in her bones and not in any of her organs. Because I had not been involved in keeping up with the status of her cancer, I knew little about how it was being managed, much less about the medications and treatments she needed. I asked a lot of questions, sometimes the same ones more than once on each visit. Momma had truly lived and dealt with this disease on her own.

My siblings and I rarely engaged in her care. Because our mom was such a strong woman and didn't ask for much, to include her care, we all perceived it as "she's good!" I never personalized the disease. Whether that's because Mom managed the treatments so well with very few side effects or just chose not to tell us. Either way, in hindsight, I feel guilty for not being more involved, for not knowing more than I did. She had been living with this disease since 2011.

The cancer went into remission in 2012 but returned in 2016. For me, my focus at first was on Clint, trying to figure out what was going on with—what we thought was—my perfectly healthy 54-year-old brother, my own kids, and my job. Mom was always "Mom" and could take care of herself or at least had her church family around to help her, and our brother Marcus was there too. My plate was full, as were those of so many people in our family, and this may also ring true for your situation.

As the saying goes, no use crying over spilled milk. I needed to be "present" for Momma now, more than ever. My primary focus when they both first moved in with me was Clint, because he had a higher need for assistance with his activities of daily living (ADLs). Mom could still function and do all her own ADLs. But I could still learn what she was dealing with, ask questions about new medications they wanted her to start or try, and inquire about the direction of her care and expectations of the disease and her quality of life. Advocate for her, and advocate I did!

Mom wanted to live life; she just did not know how to articulate or express what that looked like. She was not ready to die—she made that clear and said as much: "I don't want to die!" However, she finally opened up to me and Karla a couple of times that she was afraid of dying. Her fear was that when it happened, it would be painful or traumatic. I reminded her of who she was in Christ and where she would go when her day came. She would not say much, but the look on her face was one of doubt. Every Sunday, she would watch Pastors Robert Morris, Charles Stanley, Steven Furtick, and many others on YouTube. We tried finding a church in the area to physically attend, but so many had changed their format to watching a pastor at an alternate location on the big screen. We agreed "we can do that at home." Plus, although the music would be phenomenal, it would be excruciatingly loud. Some of the churches offered earplugs...seriously?! If a church must add earplugs to its church supply list, it might consider adjusting the volume of its worship sets. It is not a concert!

During one of Karla's visits with Mom one day, the topic of dying came up. Karla asked Mom, "What do you want?" Mom told Karla that she wanted her family around her. Karla then promised her that her kids and anyone else who could, would be by her side. Karla and I concluded that was her ultimate fear: being alone.

I imagine this to be a concern of most of the elderly population. We kept that promise when Momma's day came. I pray you too can make that same promise with your loved one.

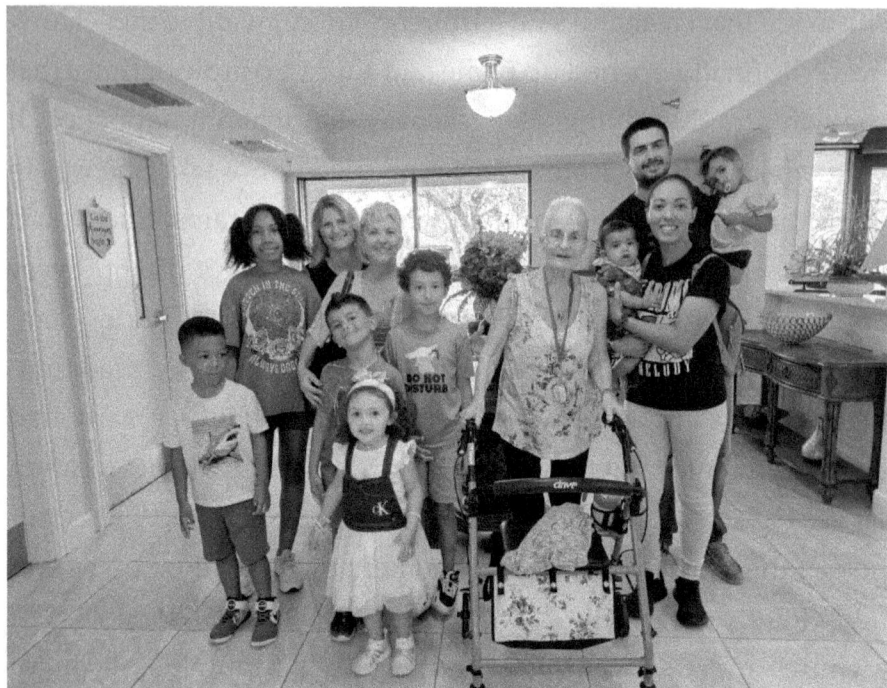

Karla, grandkids, and great-grandkids
visiting Grandma-ma, 2023

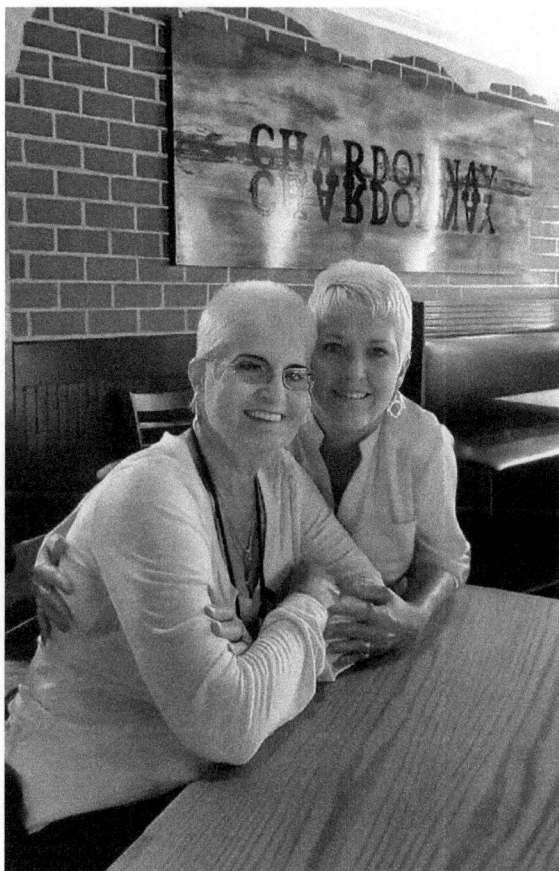

Karla and Momma at Dinner, 2022

CHAPTER THREE
ADVOCATING LIFE

Mom, the Forever Caregiver

My siblings have all lived very independent lives since becoming adults. Occasionally, we check in on each other and, if we can swing it, come together for a holiday or a family reunion. Renée remained in Florida, while Marcus lived in three different states, Clint lived in three states plus another country. And once I entered active duty in the Army, I probably moved the most, living in six states, including Florida. But for all the distance, we would try to find ways to stay close through phone calls, texting, Facebook, and the occasional family reunions.

Mom lived in Jacksonville; in the same house I grew up in just before I was born. It was not until our youngest brother Corey was around 16 years old that the rest of us decided it was time for Mom to move due to the increased crime in the area. Corey has had his challenges with the law, and when those troubles came to our mom's doorstep, all of us kids packed her up and moved her to Georgia with Marcus. She settled in quickly, attending the same church as Marcus and eventually got her own piece of land and a trailer.

Although Mom had retired from nursing, she still found herself useful to fellow church members needing the occasional "assistance" with a family member convalescing from a hospital stay. Then, when her own mother, "Grams," was officially diagnosed with Alzheimer's and her driver's license was revoked, Mom moved her in and took care of her until she passed. None of us kids really understood much about this disease called Alzheimer's, except that maybe "you forget things." When we talked to Mom about Grams, she would share some of the silly things Grams would do. These conversations with Mom about how things were going gave us all the sense that Alzheimer's was a manageable situation and that there wasn't a lot of stress. Mom would say she was doing fine, or something like, "Well, had to get Gram's today.... She walked down to the neighbor's house because she thought she was going to work. She knocked on the door and said, 'I'm here, where do you want me start?' So, the neighbor had to walk her back home." It was humorous. It wasn't something that spoke to the stress and anxiety my mom was surely experiencing or the challenges she faced daily.

Earlier in the book, I mentioned tidbits about Mom's story. After caring for her own mother, that challenge was followed by another when Marcus's wife, Janice, was diagnosed with Alzheimer's shortly after Gram passed. Mom, who found purpose in taking care of others, looked after Janice from 2011 to 2019. But Janice's experience was different from Gram's. Janice's experience with Alzheimer's not only included forgetting where things went but also experiencing high levels of anxiety and stress in random situations. One time during bath time, Janice either became unaware of her surroundings or simply felt cold and needed to "get away" or "get out." In doing so, she knocked Mom down, leaving a cut on Mom's head.

But God wasn't done teaching Mom the lessons of Job yet. While she was caring for Janice, Mom was diagnosed with breast cancer and had a lumpectomy in 2012. She went through chemo and radiation therapy, after which the cancer went into remission. We had many people praying for her, and one of my friends drove from South Carolina to Georgia just to lay hands on her and pray over her. Eventually, Mom would take one more spin as our family nurse-in-residence soon after Clint was diagnosed with FTD and could no longer live on his own. Mom took care of Clint and Janice for a short time. However, soon after moving Clint in with Mom, Janice needed the care she could only get in a medical facility. She was moved to a facility where her own daughter was the director of nursing and was able to monitor her care there and was by her side when she passed away.

Momma continued to care for others until she was 80 years old: from an LPN to private duty nurse caring for quadriplegics; her mother with Alzheimer's; her daughter-in-law with Alzheimer's; and finally, her oldest son with early-onset frontotemporal dementia —all while receiving chemotherapy and radiation therapy for stage IV breast cancer. Momma leaned on her church family the most. She also had one of her sisters, Aunt Jo-Jo (Joyce), who had moved into a rental property a few blocks down from her. Mom did a lot for Aunt Jo-Jo and her kids as they struggled to make ends meet. Aunt Jo-Jo had her own battle with cancer as well, but Mom and Jo-Jo leaned on each other as much as they could. After Aunt Jo-Jo passed away, Momma then began managing one of my cousins' (Aunt Jo-Jo's son) medical and financial affairs, because he was on disability. Mom stayed busy between her and Clint's appointments but then had to start taking my cousin to his appointments as well. Momma was a strong Christian woman: cancer didn't have a hold on her. No, Sir! She kept cancer at bay because she had people to take care of! Her son needed her and her friends at church needed her. She didn't have time for cancer!

Nonetheless, it was truly more than anyone should have to deal with or manage, much less someone in their late seventies. All of us kids knew as much when we saw her in January 2020. As much as Momma didn't want to admit it, she was tired and knew she needed a break.

Mom loved the church she belonged to in Georgia. She taught Sunday school, cooked for all the church gatherings, and volunteered for a lot of different functions at her home church. She had so many friends and just really loved participating in the ladies' groups. I know Mom never read the book entitled The Five Love Languages, but I cannot help but wonder if Acts of Service was her love language. If you have read the book, you will understand that people tend to show their love to others by acting in the way they themselves receive and recognize as love.

For example, one of my love languages is quality time. To me, when someone spends time with me, I feel loved by them (like when my dad would take me to that early breakfast before work). Before reading the book, I thought everyone felt loved when someone spent time with them. But as I learned after reading the book, quality time is not everyone's love language. Mom did not read the book, but she lived her life giving to others, caring for others. This is what brought her joy and love. I now see — or accept — that her small acts of service to me were her way of loving me, the best way she knew how.

Mom always dressed and acted like a lady. After her trailer burned down, she received boxes upon boxes of clothes and other necessities from local churches and organizations. Some of those boxes contained brand-new dresses, still with tags on them, blouses, and dress pants. Mom also loved her costume jewelry and had lots of it. She retained a lot of jewelry from her mother after she passed. She had multiple cameo pieces and a lot of pearls. Then, anytime we were out shopping at Walmart, the flea market, or stopping in at Cracker Barrel for a bite to eat, if it was sparkly and shiny, Momma just "had to have it." Our family always got a kick out of Mom's obsession with jewelry. But with her sporty white hair, shiny jewelry, and dressed to the nines, she got more compliments walking through a parking lot anywhere! She would be the best-dressed 83-year-old who looked like she was in her late 60s or early 70s, and everyone around us recognized and acknowledged it. It would put the biggest smile on her face! She especially loved it when an older gentleman would give her a compliment and open a door or pull out a chair for her. She loved chivalry. Caring for your adult child is emotionally and physically challenging, and one of her release outlets was dressing like a "lady" and receiving acknowledgment for it. Now that

I think of it, maybe words of affirmation were her second love language.

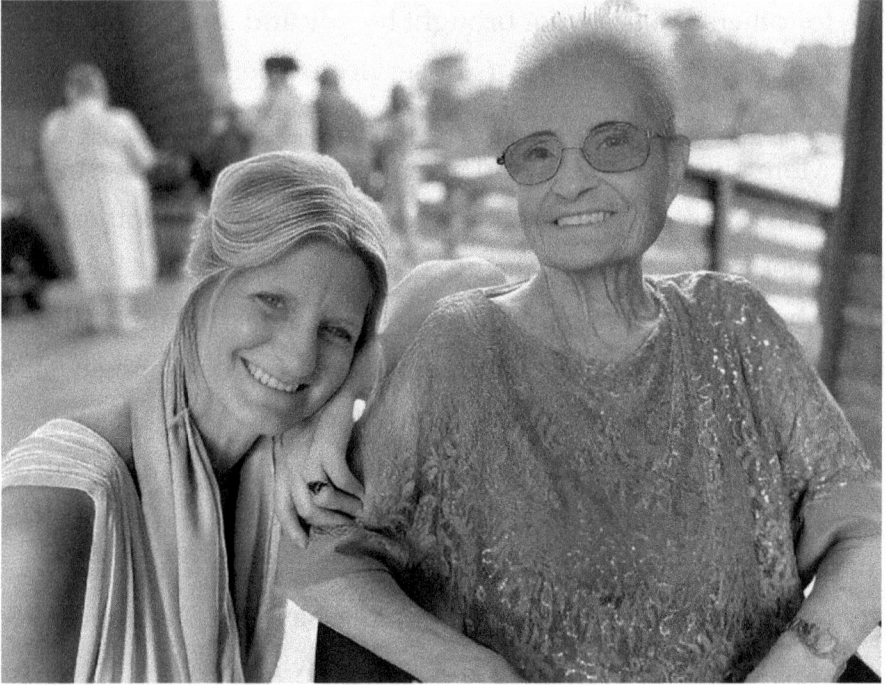

Julie and Momma at Adam's Wedding, 2022

Support Systems for You and Your Loved One

When someone is living with a disease or disability, the importance of having a support system is vital to both the person with the illness and the caregiver, affecting their recovery and outlook on life. Also known as "social support systems," Johns Hopkins Medicine defines it like this:

The persons, agencies, and organizations with which a caregiver has contact—directly or indirectly—are referred to as a person's social support system. Social support may be provided in the form of:

- *Physical or practical assistance (e.g., transportation, assistance with chores)*
- *Resource and information sharing (i.e., information on community resources)*
- *Emotional and physiological assistance (i.e., someone who listens to and encourages you)*
- *Attitude transmission (i.e., someone who helps you laugh or see things more positively)*

(https://www.hopkinsmedicine.org/about/community-health/johns-hopkins-bayview/services/called-to-care/social-support-systems)

Depending on your personality, when you first become a full-time caregiver, you may tell yourself, "I got this." That may be true for some things, but not all. When I became Mom and Clint's caregiver, I had been on a journey looking for my purpose. I had tried to enter the corporate world after giving 30 years of my life to the military. I also tried my hand at consulting and eventually got a brief gig teaching for a local university. Transitioning out of the military and back into the civilian sector is challenging. From impostor syndrome to discovering your place in the world among nonmilitary members in a functioning, contributing role to society is a challenge most military members face. But when the need presented itself for Mom and Clint's care, I saw it as a way to give them my time lost from living away from them for so long.

Full transparency, it also became a safe place for me to function without dealing with the challenges of "finding a job" or "dressing to impress." I was receiving my retirement; I didn't have a lot of bills or debt. I knew I could manage with very little assistance from their income, as well. I had learned a lot in the military, and I knew I had skills and knowledge that could serve me and them well in my duties as a caregiver. I didn't have a problem with reaching out to my family for input or advice on a given situation, but I knew there was only so much they could do. I always approached them through the lens of their limitations. Their main limitations were time: they worked 40 to 50 hours per week, cared for their grandchildren, and lived five to 10 hours away. I had no family near me to give me a break when I needed it.

My family still supported me in a different valuable way, and that was by listening. I could call either of my sisters to share a bad day I had or get their feedback on an idea I had regarding their care. That's how they supported me, Mom, and Clint.

Another way my family came together was when our dad wanted to come to Tampa to visit Clint. Daddy was no longer able to drive and lived in northern Georgia. He remarried when I was in my thirties, and he still wrote Southern gospel music and played with a band in different churches. Eventually, his wife, Elizabeth, would join him in the band, singing and playing bass guitar. They recorded a few albums together, and Daddy loved giving them away as part of his mission for God. When Daddy began developing Parkinson's, his demeanor and beliefs began to change. I now believe it was the advancing disease. Daddy changed his religion from Baptist to Seventh Day Adventist. Never in our family's history, and certainly not his wife's, had there ever been a desire to be anything but Baptist (or at least non-denominational Christian).

He became fixated on parts of the Bible that, "in context," gave a clear meaning, but out of context left you pondering. Daddy and Renée spoke often about life but mostly about the Bible. They so enjoyed discussing the love of God, and he often spoke to both of us about keeping the day of Sabbath holy. He was determined to hold everyone accountable to those who chose to work on Saturdays (a Seventh Day Adventist and Old Testament belief) and would sometimes express that belief to his wife's side of the family and their circle of friends.

Aside from preaching about the rights and wrongs of the world, Daddy loved his children and often praised each of us for our successes in life. He wanted us to visit more often than any of us did, but he would always dismiss our absence with the understanding and appreciation of each of our abilities to stand on our own two feet and sustain our lives. He often compared our successes to the young adults where he lived and shared his disapproval of their "laziness" and lack of motivation. Once again, we believed this was the disease talking as his newfound beliefs took a stronghold.

When Daddy began to get weaker and weaker, he started talking more about old times and where he grew up. I had a gut feeling that his time to leave this Earth was drawing nearer. He desperately wanted one of us kids to come get him and take him on a drive to where he lived with his parents. He called me often, knowing I cared for both Mom and Clint, and begged me to let him come live with me too. My heart ached at his request and my inability to give him what he wanted. He hadn't been able to visit with Clint in a couple of years and knew his dementia was also advancing. That's when I reached out to Marcus and Renée to put a plan in place to get Daddy to Tampa —and Daddy was excited!

Marcus drove to Daddy's and picked him up, then took him to Jacksonville to Renée's house. They spent the night with Renée, and the next day, Renée drove Daddy to my place in Tampa. Daddy and Renée stayed for a couple of days before reversing the trip to get Daddy back home. The picture below speaks for itself: the love and gratefulness our dad felt, seeing his children, especially his oldest son, one last time. The picture was taken in April 2021. Daddy passed away two months later, in June 2021.

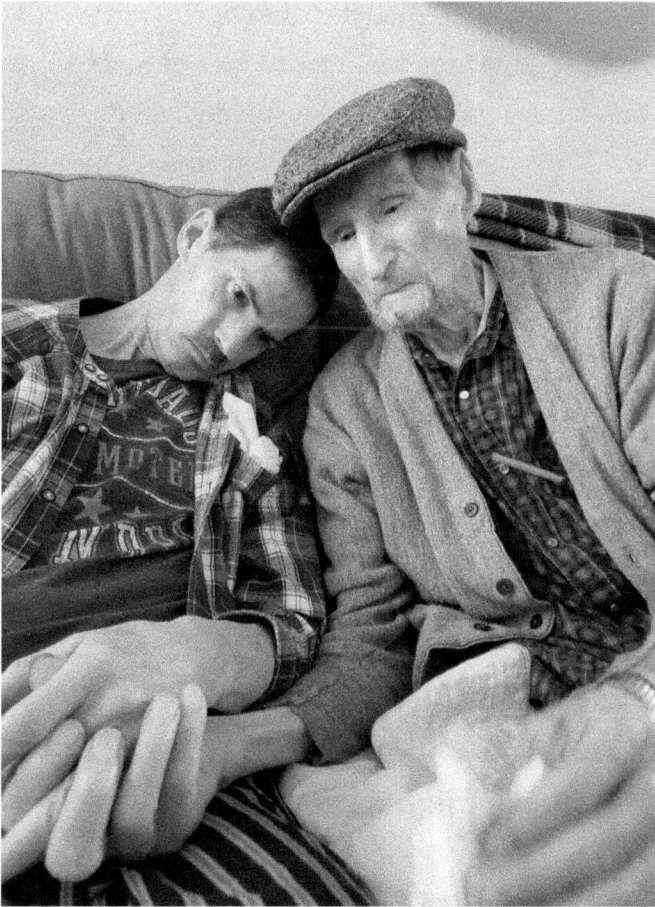
Figure 13 Daddy and Clint together one last time, 2021

Another leg of my support team included my closest friends Mike, Hope, and her sister Rachael. They themselves had gone through the struggles of caring for aging parents —one with Parkinson's, another with dementia, and another with heart problems. They were my sounding board. Anywhere they had already navigated through the various systems of medical and government agencies, they were able to share their personal experiences with me to ease my own burden of discovery, pointing me in the right direction. Not to mention offering a shoulder to lean on—or cry on. They certainly have their own story to tell, but I want to recognize them for their unwavering support and patience in hearing me unload my emotional stress.

From the Hopkins Medicine website above, it offers a brief assessment to help you review and reflect on not only who is in your support system but also helps you ask yourself hard questions, such as why some are in your support system and why some are not, or what's not working and what is working. During this assessment, you are likely to discover reasons why you haven't asked anyone for help with your situation. Start building your support team now. I would like to believe it begins with your family. However, that may not be an option for you. Reach out to organizations you belong to, such as a church. If that isn't an option, then at the very least, seek out support groups for the disease or disability afflicting the person you care for, such as the Association for Frontotemporal Dementia (www.theaftd.org) or the American Cancer Society (www.cancer.org).

Communicating with Medical Staff

Support systems also come from a group of people that I certainly expected to be a part of both Mom and Clint's support system: the doctors and nurses involved in their care. There were many individuals who were a part of each of their medical teams and who truly "showed up" with sincere care and concern for their well-being. Then there were those who were overwhelmed with their workload and struggled to pour from their empty cup.

When everyone in a support system is trying, the stress of the disease or disability seems manageable, and we all can share the burden. I grew up with the saying, "Many hands make light work!" Unfortunately, it is when someone in the chain decides "it's not my job or responsibility" that creates a weakness, if not a break in the chain. The stress of the disease or disability affects both the patient and the caregiver who is trying to manage and balance the situation and handle the rest of their lives. Without everyone in the chain contributing the same effort, the stress and burden of it all suddenly become 100 times heavier on the caregiver (family member), as well as the one being cared for.

Expectations often place us in frustrating situations. *Psychology Today* states, "It is the attachment to those expectations [that] is the source of our suffering" (https://www.psychologytoday.com/us/blog/the-wisdom-of-anger/202309/how-to-manage-expectations). My expectations for the doctors and nurses caring for both my brother and mother sometimes exceeded reality.

Navigating the healthcare system continues to be a challenge for everyone. Every hospital, every medical practice, every governmental agency has its own process and standards. If managing someone's expectations can be included in some of those processes, I would hope it could bring better communication between the family, medical staff, and the governmental agencies involved.

I would venture to say most people don't plan to live with a terminal disease. When families are hit by these unexpected diagnoses, having a system in place to orient the individual and their families to what is expected would be helpful. This process is no different from onboarding as a new employee: being required to sit through an orientation to the company you are working for and learning about the benefits of the job, as well as what your new role will entail. What if hospitals or private practices offered an orientation class on the terminal disease you have been diagnosed with?

For now, we are given a brochure to read or a website to go to and figure out on our own what to expect. I realize our society, within all industries, has shifted to this model of education (watch this video and teach yourself). But when you are dealing with a stressful diagnosis of an early death, I personally would rather have a little handholding and the personal touch of reassurance that there is a system in place to help me get through this difficult time. This yearning was my attachment to the expectations I had with medical staff and what added to my own suffering and anxiety.

During my time in the military, I learned to become a person who doesn't like to mince words. As I've mentioned earlier, I have found it better to be direct and straight to the point in an effort to save time and energy. Sometimes I show more finesse in my delivery, but there are times I will be more assertive to either shake someone from their narrow view on a situation or to simply express my understanding and seek answers to what I may be misunderstanding. Just as I found myself in this predicament with my brother and some of his medical team, the scenario would repeat itself when my mother was hospitalized. Communicating with medical staff as an advocate for your loved one is necessary.

You should not just assume that medical personnel will always have the right answers and that your job is to sit back and never question their decisions. Advocating for another human being means you are questioning every decision being made for their well-being. If something doesn't seem right, go with your gut and ask questions. I did exactly that!

End of Chapter Takeaways

Some key takeaways, I hope you see, include recognizing your loved one's purpose in life. When you pay attention to what brings joy or a smile to their face and you take the time to give that back to them—even for a moment—it will bring you the joy you've been seeking. Doing so, no matter how big or small the act, will fill your "love bank account" more than you can imagine.

This chapter also covers the value and importance of having support around you. That support hopefully will come from your family, friends, and any organization you belong to, whether it's a faith-based or religious group or even a business organization. You need these support channels to help you emotionally, physically, and mentally. This chapter also discussed the importance of open communication with the medical teams in charge of your loved one's healthcare. You need to have the courage to speak up, ask hard questions, and seek answers to what doesn't make sense to you.

CHAPTER FOUR
THE STRENGTH OF YOUR VOICE

Setting Expectations

When we moved back to the Jacksonville area to be close to family and friends that Mom still had in the area, I had to find all new doctors for Mom and me. I was still looking after Clint, who had initially been placed in an assisted living facility until he was able to be admitted into a VA home for all his care.

Mom's oncologist, Dr. K., was very personable, compassionate, and aware of Mom's needs. Dr. K. also ensured that Mom received information for any financial assistance she needed to help with the cost of medication, such as applying to the manufacturer to receive a discount based on income. That same oncologist also educated us on what all Medicare would cover. Mom's oncologist in Jacksonville was probably the best and most attentive she had had during her history of cancer. Dr. K. also gave me her cell number so I could let her know when Mom was showing signs of a UTI, a common recurrence for the elderly, especially with cancer treatments, so Mom could get in for testing, IV fluids, and the right prescription. This doctor, I truly believe, advocated for Mom. I have often felt as though those doctors are few and far between, especially in a larger metro area.

Chemotherapy and radiation therapy are double-edged swords. They attack the cancer cells, shrinking them down, but they also destroy the good cells and weaken the immune system. Mom had been on and off both for many years. We sought out a couple of natural remedies to try to help with strengthening her immune system again, particularly turkey tail mushrooms. There is a great video by the well-known scientist Paul Stamets, who has studied multiple types of mushrooms and their health benefits. Here is a link to a speaking engagement he did with Next Med Health, conducted about eight years ago:

https://www.youtube.com/watch?v=7agK0nkiZpA&t=684s.

Momma did incorporate some of the mushrooms recommended by Mr. Stamets; however, without the proper professional guidance from a physician who was educated in this line of defense against cancer, our efforts did not show any significant results, and she stopped using them.

Mom was doing very well with the chemotherapy she was receiving. Her strength and energy were better, and she enjoyed sitting on the back patio in the fresh air, going to the pool, and taking walks around the neighborhood. She reconnected with her closest friend, Ada, who she used to attend church with when she lived in Jacksonville. Ada and Mom were able to spend time together and went out to lunch on at least one occasion that I recall. Ada would also come to our house to spend time with Mom, and Mom loved it! Being close to family and one of her closest friends lifted Mom's spirits.

Mom has two sisters who live in Florida, and we made plans for her to visit the one in the panhandle so Charles and I could take a trip to visit our kids. My aunt was briefed (if you will) on Mom's routines and medications, and I showed her all the insurance information, in the event of an emergency. No different from leaving your small children with a babysitter, I had to do the same with my mom. The day prior to Charles and I traveling home, I received a text from my aunt that Mom wasn't feeling well. We had been gone only about three days by then. Mom had had a round of radiation prior to our trip. Everything my aunt was telling me was pointing to signs that she needed to get to an ER. But my aunt, even though this was her sister, was not familiar with Mom's routines or behaviors and wasn't sure how to interpret what she was witnessing. This was a lesson learned for us: even though Momma was with another family member, they won't always fully understand the gravity of the level of care that the person with a disease or disability requires. I know I did my best to inform my aunt and prepare her for potential emergency situations. The rest was up to my aunt, if nothing else, to lean on her own parenting skills and life experiences to decide what to do in case of an emergency. Nonetheless, I can only surmise that my aunt leaned more into the notion that her sister was a grown woman, capable of telling someone she needed to go to the hospital, instead of watching for the subtle cues of illness that fall outside of normal behavior. My mom and aunt had not spent a lot of time around each other in many years, so to her defense, she didn't really know what "normal" looked like. I suppose my aunt truly did not see the storm that was brewing inside my mom.

The final decision came when my aunt sent me a picture of Mom's face as I was standing in the airport, which she described as "a little swollen." When I saw that picture, however, it was much worse! Mom was almost unrecognizable as she now looked like a blowfish. One side of her face was so swollen her eyes were nearly black and blue and swollen shut. EMS was called. Mom's parotid glands (a.k.a. salivary glands) had become blocked, causing a severe infection. By the time she was admitted to ICU, tested, and diagnosed (nearly twelve hours after arriving at the ER), she had become septic. I believe this was a direct result of the radiation therapy she had for the tumors sitting between her skull and brain and part of her neck, and quite possibly the new chemotherapy she was receiving.

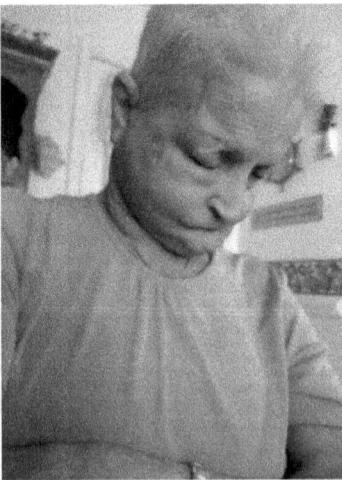

Picture of Mom's face showing infection, 2022

The website https://www.cancer.gov/about-cancer/treat-ment/side-effects/mouth-throat states, "Cancer treatments may cause mouth, throat, and dental problems. Radiation therapy to the head and neck may harm the salivary glands and tissues in your mouth and/or make it hard to chew and swallow safely. Some types of chemotherapy and immunotherapy can also harm cells in your mouth, throat, and lips. Drugs used to treat cancer and certain bone problems may also cause oral problems."

Were we made aware of the different side effects? Yes. We received a pamphlet of information, but there is no way of knowing how anyone will respond to the therapy. Mom, being "Mom," had energy, was excited about taking a road trip, and spending time with her sister. On all fronts, she was having a great response to the therapy. Until she didn't. She spent eighteen days in the hospital near my aunt's home.

Once in the ICU, the pressure of being Mom's medical surrogate was soon realized as she lay unconscious. Since we were away from home, away from her regular doctors and medical records, when the MRI showed multiple tumors on her brain, they called in a neurosurgeon to talk to me about surgery and the possibility of the tumors being cancerous. The surgeon was emphasizing the urgency of the matter, and rightfully so. However, what was new information for her was old news to me.

I tried to explain to the surgeon Momma's medical history, that she was under the care of an oncologist, and we were fully aware of the tumors. I also contacted Mom's oncologist and requested the two speak to each other to compare notes and come to a logical or practical solution. However, that did not stop the

ICU doctor or the hospital oncologist from basically telling me that my mother was on her deathbed, and I needed to start facing the decision to sign a DNR (Do Not Resuscitate) form. Initially I did sign it, but after speaking with Mom's oncologist at home and a friend who is an ICU nurse on how to make that decision, I canceled the DNR almost as fast as I signed it.

Momma wasn't ready to die, nor were we ready to let her go. Momma's oncologist knew her cancer was in a stable state—enough so that it communicated to me that Momma still had many months of life to live. All in all, her oncologist and my ICU nurse friend assured me that the decision was absolutely mine to make. In making that *life-or-death* decision, however, I wanted—needed—to have *all* the facts. That included Mom's wishes. Weighing what my mother wanted with her potential outcomes while also listening to the voices of the doctors and surgeons standing directly in front of me was enough to set off my anxiety. Anyone's anxiety! But I remained steadfast. *"I AM HER VOICE!"* I reminded myself. I thanked the neurosurgeon, hospital oncologist, and ICU doctor for their input, but this was my decision, and they needed to do whatever needed to be done to help Momma fight this infection. I asked them for alternative options.

Momma was fighting an infection in her body, but her immune system wasn't quite strong enough. I pointed out that she had spent nearly 12 hours in the ER without food or water as the staff waited for test results. I further noted that she had been on antibiotics since arriving at the ICU and, after nearly 24 hours, began showing signs of improvement as the swelling in her face was reducing. The doctor agreed she was improving enough to be released from the ICU, and they moved her to a regular room in the hospital. Once there, the attending physician (I'll call him "Dr. A" for 'amazing') recommended Mom be given a total parenteral nutrition (TPN) line. She was still unconscious, unable to have anything by mouth, but needed to start receiving some form of nutrition to help her body begin the process of strengthening. The attending and I had a very thorough and thoughtful conversation about either surgically inserting a feeding tube in her stomach or doing the TPN for 3–5 days, in hopes of her waking and starting to eat on her own. Momma really was not a candidate for any surgery, not to mention she had made it very clear in her Advanced Healthcare Directive that, should the time arise for a feeding tube, her decision was to seek alternatives and not to have one placed. Therefore, TPN was administered. Dr. A helped me advocate for my mom.

Mom continued with a cocktail of antibiotics and low doses of morphine to manage any pain. A neurologist had come to evaluate Mom after she was assigned to a room. He tried to wake her, but to no avail. He recommended taking her off the morphine in hopes of waking her up, and by day three, when he came in to try and stir her, her eyes opened. The neurologist smiled and looked at me and said, "This is progress!" At which point he felt she was on the mend and basically discharged her from his (specialty) care.

Momma couldn't talk yet, and a speech pathologist was assigned to work with her and control her diet, starting with a liquid-only diet. By day five, the TPN was stopped and a soft food diet, like applesauce and yogurt, was started. Momma still wasn't talking much, but she would nod her head when you asked her questions. The physician was very transparent, communicating, and discussing Mom's care and options with me. I immediately shared the family's desire to get her released to either another hospital or rehabilitation center in Jacksonville, closer to our home. A case manager was assigned to Mom to help begin discussions about when she was ready to be discharged, depending on her needs when that day came.

Within the first two days of being admitted to a regular room, three different case managers were "assigned" to Mom's case. She eventually ended up having a fourth, and that was the last one she had. This, in and of itself, was very frustrating. Having to constantly reiterate her needs and the plans to move her became exhausting with everything else going on. On her third day in her room, a new attending physician came on shift. I'll call him "Dr. V" (for "vulture"). He was her doctor for the rest of her stay, and he was neither compassionate nor transparent. I had shared with Dr. V the family's wish to have Mom moved to a facility that was closer to home as soon as she was stable enough to either ride in my car or, if need be, via ambulance. From the moment he entered her room when he came on shift, and every day he came in to check off his blocks of evaluation, his mind was made up that (1) Mom needed to be in hospice care and (2) she was not leaving this hospital.

When Mom was awake, alert, and able to say a few words (roughly around day five or six), Dr. V entered her room for his daily checks. I asked him again about having Mom moved to another facility closer to our home. He blurted out that "insurance is not likely to approve Mom being moved, especially since she should be on hospice." Mom heard him say this and she looked at him and adamantly yelled out, "NO!" For a patient who, according to Dr. V, "wasn't showing improvement or progress" and "needed to be under hospice care because she is going to die," she had enough strength and wits about her to immediately put this doctor in his place. She yelled so loud it even startled me. But I grinned, looked at the doctor, and reiterated, "I'll get with the case manager to begin planning her discharge."

I continued my efforts to have Mom transferred, but Dr. V continued to circumvent those efforts and avert our plans. After Mom expressed her opposition to hospice care, Dr. V would agree that Mom was showing improvement, stating in front of me and the case worker that Mom was eligible to transfer to a long-term acute care facility (LTAC). Mom was eating by mouth on her own, and physical therapy was able to get her up and walking. The speech pathologist was delaying her diet change to solid foods, so when I saw Momma frown at the mushy food, they were trying to feed her, I asked, "Momma, are you hungry for something else?" She just sort of shrugged. I asked, "Would you like me to get you a chicken sandwich or hamburger?" At first, she seemed undecided or unsure of what to say or do. My family knows me to be direct. I was dealing with a doctor ready to hammer the nail in my mother's coffin while I was trying to do my due diligence as her medical surrogate. I said, "Momma, you need to get stronger. Eating and getting nourishment will help you do that." I then asked, "Are you ready to die? If you are, tell me now." She hesitated, looked down at the puréed food on her plate, looked at me, and said, "I want a hamburger." So, I went to the cafeteria and bought her a hamburger and fries. She nearly ate the whole plate! The nurse was surprised to see her eating so well. I asked the nurse to please send a message to the speech pathologist that she was ready for solid food. It took nearly twenty-four hours to get the order in the system, so the next day I went to Cracker Barrel and bought her some chicken and dumplings with green beans and a sweet tea!

Momma continued to get stronger and talk more. The case manager contacted the facility Momma was going to be transferred to, as they had to first agree to accept Mom before insurance was contacted. Once that acceptance came, the caseworker began the process of getting insurance authorization. By this time, Dr. V returned to his tactics of deceit, stating that insurance was not likely to approve the move because Mom was not improving, and she belonged in hospice care. His insatiable tactics to keep her in that hospital became more and more prevalent. I stopped him in his tracks, refusing to accept his prognosis.

I reminded him of just how much Mom had improved and progressed over the last week and a half: from being weaned off the TPN, to the swelling going down, to waking up, talking, and now walking and eating by mouth. Unfortunately, the seed had been planted, as he apparently made this note in her records. After every shift, when a new nurse came on the floor, they would pull me aside and whisper in my ear, "You know, I've seen this numerous times. When a patient like your mom has been through something like this or has dreams or visions of past relatives (of which Mom recalls seeing her deceased sister while she was unconscious), then you need to start preparing yourself for their passing." I was almost strangely calm when I responded after the second nurse said this to me. I asked, "Is there something in her chart that says she is about to die?" The nurse confirmed that Dr. V listed in his notes that the patient needed to be placed in hospice and not expected to make it. I vehemently, firmly, looked that nurse square in her eyes and said, "Let me tell you something: my mother has made significant improvements over the last few days. Enough improvement that tells me she is not ready to die. So do me, my family, and yourself a favor and remove that statement from my mother's records and inform your colleagues! The next staff member to tell me that my mother needs to be on hospice or that she is about to die will be removed from my mother's case. Am I clear?!"

My mother came to the ER on May 16th, and by May 25th, before the insurance company would grant the authorization for Mom to be moved to an LTAC, the insurance company's chief medical officer (CMO) needed to have a peer-to-peer meeting with the attending physician, Dr. V. That meeting took place on May 27th, and afterward, Dr. V. came into my mother's room, his chest puffed up, to inform us that "the insurance" denied the request for transfer, stating that she did not meet the requirements because she was on antibiotics and TPN for ten or more days. I corrected the doctor that, although she was still on antibiotics, she wasn't on the cocktail she was initially on and that the TPN was stopped at day five—and (again) she *was* having signs of progress and improvement. Dr. V. made these statements in front of the case manager, as well. No sooner did Dr. V. give that information, he then stated, "It's how insurance companies operate now; something to do with reserving resources or saving money." I interpreted this last statement to mean my mother's life was not worthy of a chance for survival and she was being advised to accept her demise and seek hospice as her only option. Dr. V. then turned around and walked out.

The case manager and I walked back to his office to call the insurance company and seek alternatives, as well as look into having her transferred to maybe a rehabilitation center near our home. The insurance company had also assigned a case manager, and that is who we called and put on speaker.

The insurance case manager was reviewing the notes from the peer-to-peer review with Dr. V. and their CMO and made the comment that it was the attending physician who *withdrew the request* for my mother to be transferred to LTAC. Both the hospital case manager and I looked at each other in total shock! We asked the insurance case manager to repeat those words. So, I specifically asked her, "Are you saying your CMO did NOT deny my request?" The insurance case manager confirmed that. She reiterated that Dr. V. withdrew the request. I was LIVID! I went directly to the hospital administrator's office and demanded Dr. V. be removed from my mother's case and an investigation be done. This was a blatant violation of my mother's rights.

I also wrote a letter to the hospital's chief medical officer, stating the following:

Looking over the patient rights listed on your hospital's website and the ethics and responsibilities of physicians on the AMA website I feel as though my mother's rights were violated and treatment withheld for the following reasons:

1. *The attending physician, Dr. V., violated multiple principles of medical ethics to include:*
   a. *failure to uphold the standards of professionalism; honesty in all professional interactions, and he engaged in acts of deception.*
   b. *failure to regard responsibility to the patient as paramount.*
   c. *failure to support access to medical care for all people.*
2. *The attending physician, Dr. V., violated the AMA Code of Medical Ethics Opinion 1.1.3 to include:*
   a. *failure to provide the patient's right to courtesy, respect, dignity, and timely, responsive attention to his or her needs.*
   b. *failure to provide guidance about what they consider the optimal course of action for the patient based on the physician's objective professional judgment.*
   c. *failure to allow the patient to ask questions about their health status or recommended treatment when they do not fully understand what has been described and to have their questions answered.*
   d. *failure to make decisions about the care the physician recommends and to have those decisions respected.*
   e. *failure to be advised of any conflicts of interest their physician may have in respect to their care.*
   f. *failure to respect the rights of patients to continuity of care.*

3. *The attending physician, Dr. V., violated the AMA Code of Medical Ethics Opinion 1.1.8 by failing to collaborate in a discharge plan that was determined safe. Instead, Dr. V. impeded the process of a proper and safe discharge and transfer through deception and dishonesty.*

It was on a Friday afternoon at 3:00 p.m. when I received the notice that Mom was stable enough to transport her to a rehab facility close to our home in my car. Our case manager was out, and his replacement did nothing but complain that my mother's Medicare Advantage Plan was too complicated and I should seriously consider switching her to the regular Medicare plan because it was easier for her to do her job.

Then, since it was so late in the day (she didn't get off work for another two hours), we would have to wait until the following week to finish the discharge paperwork. It was Memorial Day weekend, and for no other reason than that, my mother was forced to remain in the hospital for an additional seven days. She was finally discharged into my care on June 3rd. This incident was also included in my letter to the CMO, reminding him that it is not the case manager's job to inform patients or their families what insurance plans they should have to make their job easier.

To say I was vehemently appalled at all we had to deal with is an understatement. The patient was no longer the center of concern. Money, selfishness, and self-aggrandizement became the clear focus of their culture. I did receive a personal phone call from the hospital's CMO to offer an apology for the poor decisions made by Dr. V. and some of the staff. Although he could not divulge any details, he assured me an investigation was initiated.

I don't want to mislead you when it comes to the decision to transition to hospice care. At this point, we knew it wasn't time. But in the back of my mind, I knew there would come a day when that decision would need to be made, and I needed to be ready to make that decision, especially as her medical surrogate.

The Beginning of Mom's Decline

Mom left that hospital and within a few months, she began having back-to-back UTIs, hence her doctor giving me the "bat phone" number to call when symptoms started. I had to ensure she was staying hydrated. It took nearly two years of her living with me and my pushing that narrative of "drink more water," but she finally did start loving to drink water. She reached the point of asking for it often on her own.

Urinary tract infections are no joke for the elderly. They throw their mental state into a loop, presenting symptoms of advanced stages of dementia. After getting Mom home from her sister's—an 18-day stay in the hospital and a one-week stay at a rehabilitation center close to home—she was still a little weak. I kept a close eye on her every move. If she went to the bathroom, I was at the door. When she needed to bathe, I had a shower chair for her and helped her bathe, mostly for physical support. Until one morning, we were getting ready for her doctor's appointment. I took her to the bathroom and decided to close the door to give her privacy. She tried to get dressed on her own and lost her balance, fell, and broke the head of her femur bone, which connected to the hip. EMS was called, and she was taken to the ER for x-rays to confirm the break.

She was moved to another hospital downtown, where the only surgeon available could operate. Mom was in so much pain, and I sat with her until it was time for her to go into surgery—however, nearly twelve hours later.

For twelve hours I sat with Momma as she screamed in pain. They had given her as much morphine as they were allowed to, and I think at one point they gave her Haldol to allow her some rest. After surgery, when Momma began waking up, she was very confused. It reminded me of when she would get UTIs, but this was worse. She didn't want to cooperate with the nurses or physical therapists when they came in. I began researching the effects of anesthesia in the elderly and quickly learned that confusion was considered common.

Day two after her hip surgery, I was waiting for the attending physician to drop by. It wasn't until the evening when he got to her room. I pulled him outside to discuss Mom's behavior, and at first, he began asking me questions about her mental state prior to surgery. I assured him she showed zero signs of dementia, to which he was alluding.

I then asked him about the side effects of anesthesia in the elderly, plus the amount of pain medication that was already on board prior to the surgery. He paused, stating, "You're right, anesthesia in the elderly can present dementia-like behavior." He agreed to make a note of that and give her more time to recover.

I was honestly beside myself. Why am I, a non-medical person, having to conduct differentials with a doctor about my mom's (or even Clint's) medical status? But once again I was quickly reminded, "I am (truly) their voice."

This doctor was prepared to write in her chart, diagnosing her with a disease that would not only follow her in her future care but take away the focus of her progress and recommend she be transferred to a nursing home. Within a few days she was discharged to a rehabilitation facility.

The rehab facility was located on the St. Johns River, a beautiful place. They offered Mom great care, and she loved being able to go outside to enjoy the sun and sit by the water. Mom was improving quickly as she got herself up every morning, into her wheelchair, and she would go down to the physical therapy room before they had a chance to come to her. The staff enjoyed Mom's enthusiasm and smile and her desire to get herself up, dressed, and put on makeup every day. This was not a woman drifting into the demise of dementia or even hospice. This was a woman with a new outlook on life. She left that rehab in a wheelchair, and within about two months, was using a walker. Mom was in better spirits.

Although we were enjoying being closer to family and friends, I found myself yearning for more time with my siblings, then realizing I had lived away for far too long to rekindle some friendships no matter how hard I tried. Everyone had grown, not necessarily "apart," but just into their own routines. I mean, if any of us ever needed help, we would all come together because that's what families do, or should do, for each other. However, everyone had their own circle of friendships and suddenly I didn't feel at home any longer. Even Mom's sister, who lived nearby, declined to visit or have Mom over for a visit. I considered the reasons I chose to move away at 18, which included finding success in both career and family life. Both of which I found. Then the reasons for moving back were to get Mom closer to family and coordinating time together became more and more challenging.

I also left because I wanted to get away from the pains of poverty and crime that perforated the neighborhood, I grew up in. Many of my friends either still lived in those neighborhoods or they had attachments there. The home that Mom and I moved into just outside of Jacksonville was in a great neighborhood. However, soon after moving in, I began seeing that crime line creep closer and closer. I wasn't equipped to manage caring for Mom and Clint if crime knocked on our door. I was also hoping for more family barbecues; however, my siblings were dealing with their own life routines or crises. Within about 18 months of buying and moving into this brand-new home, I began questioning why I had moved back to where I grew up and suddenly desired to move.

Charles and I talked about moving, and we both wanted to be back on the Gulf side of the state. Mom was still recovering, but as soon as she was strong enough, I shared with her our thoughts on moving again. She wasn't keen on the idea of moving so soon, but she understood. She so enjoyed it when my siblings, niece, and nephew and their kids came over. She loved having a houseful of family members, especially the kids. My niece would come over with her kids to see "Grandma-ma," and Mom would love on them or go to the pool. My niece has five children, so whenever there was a birthday, she would throw the best parties and we both loved being a part of that. Unfortunately, that wasn't enough for me to stay. I could not find, nor did I get a sense of growth if I remained in Jacksonville. Too many old memories. Had either of my siblings had the space or ability to take Mom in, they would have. So, we moved.

We sold my house and, with Mom and her dog, Charlie, moved to a condo in the Fort Myers area. We were there almost two months when Hurricane Ian hit. The morning of the storm, when it came ashore as category five, we packed up Charles's car and headed north to some friends in Lake City. We fared okay from the storm —granted, we had just moved, so the garage was still filled with boxes. The garage and back lanai had taken on water from Ian, and we had to throw out a lot of the items in those boxes. But we chose to accept it as nature's way of helping us decide what to get rid of. We were moving from a 2,400-square-foot home to an 1,100-square-foot home. What could possibly be saved was eventually given away to others who were now in desperate need due to the storm. Everything worked out as it needed to. Although, I didn't feel so giving at the time.

My anxiety reached levels I had never experienced, and I needed help. Being a full-time caregiver to both of my family members and dealing with both of their hospitalizations, going through a divorce, moving multiple times in a two-year period, reconnecting and remarrying my husband, and now dealing with the aftermath of a category five hurricane, my cup was dry, and I had nothing more to give. I cried almost every day. I wasn't sleeping, barely getting three hours of sleep per day, and my body weight began to accumulate quickly, gaining nearly 20 pounds in about a four-month span. To this day, I am still struggling with my weight, but I was able to get the care I needed.

I had started seeing a therapist prior to getting back into a relationship with my husband. But after the hurricane, I sought out care from the VA mental health clinic. I shared with the psychiatrist my disagreement with getting on medication but was open to something natural, or at least non-addictive and non-sedative. I had a history of mild depression back in my thirties and was prescribed Wellbutrin. I was on that medication for the entirety of my thirties and chose to stop it around the age of 42. I remembered how numbing the antidepressant made me feel and how little I remembered during that decade of my life. I didn't want to be numb again.

The psychiatrist suggested a medication that I would have to order on my own, as the VA did not carry it, nor would they pay for it. I began taking L-theanine to ease my anxiety, and it worked. I have been able to stop taking it and reintroduce it as needed. I continue to see a therapist as needed, but usually once a month, sometimes every two months. My coping skills have gotten better, and having my husband's and closest friends' support has been immeasurable. When's the last time you did a self-evaluation? What are you struggling with? If you are a caregiver but not seeing a therapist, I want to encourage you to. Look into something called "respite" care in your area. That is where local senior living facilities will allow you to check your loved ones into their facility for a short stay, like a week (each facility is different). If you do not have the support of family or friends to take over your shift to allow you to rest, research respite care as an option. You need your rest too! Otherwise, you will find yourself pouring from an empty cup like I was. I will tell you also the service is not free, although there are government agencies that will assist with the cost, if not pay for it in full.

I wonder if Mom had become depressed as well. We no longer lived near family and friends, and once again she moved. I've also wondered if she had a near-death experience (NDE) during that first hospital stay near her sister. She did tell me that Aunt Joyce (deceased) visited her on a couple of occasions. I wonder if during either of her hospital stays, maybe she got a chance to not only see her loved ones that passed before her but experience the energy and love of Heaven. Maybe she experienced not being in pain, then reentering her body and feeling all the pain again. Maybe she also experienced the deep emotions of love that she never experienced or expressed while on this Earth. And, if so, she was sad about being caught between two realities: wanting to be here with her family but also wanting to be in a world pain-free and full of love and high energy. I began watching documentaries on people that had NDEs, and these same experiences were shared repeatedly. The more I learned of people's experiences of love and pure energy beyond life on this Earth, the more intrigued I became with Mom's experience and the potential of my own, when that day comes.

Not able to express her emotions very well, I tried my best to keep Mom active, encouraging her to take walks and not allow her hips to lock up. But the pressure of being her entertainment guide only increased my own anxiety. I knew she did not want to go to a senior living facility, but considering her own emotional outlook on life—sitting in front of a TV all day and all night, not moving—was not healthy. I began suggesting the idea to her in an effort for her to meet people her age and to get involved with activities. We did find a great place in Fort Myers and were able to get her moved just before Christmas 2022. My family and I all wish we could have gotten her into a facility like this sooner. She soon became the center of attention, being the classy woman she was—from the way she dressed to her accessories.

During mealtimes, they had a dining room set up like a restaurant, and she was assigned to a table with nothing but men! (Oh boy!) Of course, the men doted on her and she loved it. She enjoyed going outside to soak up the sunlight and take walks. She was still using her walker, as she still had a lot of pain in the leg/hip she broke. Unfortunately, starting in January 2023, the UTIs increased, which meant more trips to the hospital. I was called on each of those visits, and I would meet her in the ER and stay until she was placed in a room, sometimes waiting six to eight hours in the ER. One time she had to use the bathroom so badly, no one was available to assist her to the bathroom. A nurse put up a divider and gave me a bedpan to help her relieve herself while lying on the gurney.

By the end of January, tests showed the cancer had spread to her liver, and this time, we knew it was time for hospice. Mom was still in fear of dying and didn't want to sign a DNR. The hospice doctor gently explained to Mom and me that, with Mom weighing barely 115 pounds and her bones already fragile from the cancer, should she have a medical event requiring CPR, her ribs would break. Recovering from broken ribs would be just as traumatic and extremely painful. Momma finally conceded and signed the DNR.

My brother Marcus had been living with us, working with Charles in his business. We stepped up our efforts of spending time with Mom, taking her to her favorite restaurant, Olive Garden. Just a block down from her senior living facility was an Olive Garden. I still would drive over to take her to all her appointments, or grocery shopping, or to get our nails done, and we would always make a point to stop at Olive Garden, if not some other place to grab lunch. A few times I came over to the facility when they would have events. About mid-to-late March, they had Disco Day. The activities director had disco décor and played a variety of dance music. Mom had these big disco glasses on, and I have a video of her dancing away. We both had a lot of fun. The nurses at her facility backed off some in monitoring her care, as a hospice nurse would do weekly checks on her. All in all, Mom was doing well. I think about one week after Disco Day was Easter Sunday. Charles, Marcus, and I went over to see Mom. We hung out in the courtyard area eating chocolate bunnies and other treats. I brought bunny ears for Mom to wear.

The next day, Monday, Mom called to ask me to bring her more water bottles. She had been drinking lots and lots of water. I told her I would bring some over the following morning, as I needed to run to Walmart. Tuesday when I came over, she was very tired and lying in bed. I sat next to her and just held her hand. She talked a little bit but then drifted off to sleep. I turned on some Southern gospel music on her TV and sat praying for about twenty minutes. A prayer I had come to repeat for the last few months. Knowing Mom's fears about dying and knowing the possibility of my Aunt Jo-Jo's spirit being there, I would ask Aunt Jo-Jo and God that when Momma's time came, let it be a peaceful experience. Over and over, I would pray that prayer. I made sure Momma was comfortable and her music was playing, kissed her on the forehead, and left.

It was close to lunchtime when I left Mom's room, so I decided to see what restaurants were around. Ruby Tuesdays popped up, and I had not been to one in over a year. I love their salad bar and thought, *Perfect!* As I began the drive over, something odd happened. As if someone were sitting beside me, I got the strongest whiff of fresh lemons squeezed into my nose. I looked around and said, "Whoa! What was that about?!" Curious, and doubtful, I looked to see if there were cars around me or maybe someone with a lemonade stand, thinking that maybe the scent came through my vents. Nothing. There were no cars around me and no lemons to speak of. I began questioning the meaning of it. Questioning if it was a sign that Momma was about to pass away. Did Momma like lemons? Sure, she did. But what was smelling lemons supposed to mean?

I arrived at Ruby Tuesday's, and the moment I stepped into the doorway, the connection to the lemons was evident. Sitting on the hostess stand was a bucket with a sign stating that they were taking collections for children with leukemia. The connection, however, was behind the hostess stand. It was a large poster board where someone had drawn pictures of lemons. The picture on the bucket was of a child with leukemia and more pictures of lemons. I immediately said, "Ok! I got the message!" I donated and went on with my lunch.

Later that afternoon, Momma called me because she had been trying to put the foot pedals back onto her wheelchair (she had become too weak to use her walker). She had fallen recently, and I reminded her that the necklace around her neck had a call button and that she needed to let the nurse do that. Mom, being "mom," said, "I know, I just wanted to try." I made her sit on the bed and push the button. I asked her to tell me when the red light was flashing. She did. I said, "Okay, now just wait for the nurse to come in and help." She said, "OK" and told me, "Good night." As a reminder, Mom didn't always show affection, but something nudged me, telling me to "say it!—tell her!" Before I hung up, I said, "I love you, Mom!" She told me back, "I love you, too." That was the last time we spoke.

The next morning, on Wednesday, I was preparing to attend a luncheon with the local Chamber of Commerce. Around 10 a.m., Mom's hospice nurse called. She said Mom had begun transitioning and I needed to come right away. I didn't understand what she meant. The nurse explained that when Mom didn't show up for breakfast, the nurses came to check on her and were unable to wake her. She was still breathing on her own, but she was in a very deep sleep. The hospice nurse further explained that when someone is about to die, they go through a transitioning phase as their body begins to shut down. My heart began pounding. My mind immediately flashed back over the last few days, especially the day prior, with my experience with the lemons. I felt lost. I wasn't ready. Was she ready? Is this it? Is Momma about to die, right now?!

I called Marcus and Charles first so they could meet me in Mom's room. I then called Renée and Karla. Karla immediately began making plans to drive down. Renée felt she couldn't take off from work and was hopeful that Mom would be okay, unsure if this was "it." She asked me to call her when I got to Mom so she could talk to her over the speakerphone. I canceled my luncheon and drove over to Mom's.

When I arrived, she looked like she was peacefully sleeping. Marcus, Charles, and I sat with her for the remainder of the day. During that time, I asked the facility nurses, "What happens next?" I asked about turning Mom and changing her as she began to sweat, but the nurses were either not available or not allowed to do anything since she was under the care of hospice. I eventually called the hospice nurse, who strongly recommended we move Mom to a hospice house, since the facility was not equipped (skilled/otherwise) to manage Mom during her transition. I knew there was one close to my home and made the necessary arrangements to move her that evening. Fortunately, they had a bed for Mom.

Karla arrived that evening, and with her and I sitting in the two available recliners, Marcus found a spot on the floor, and we stayed with Mom during her time at the hospice house. The hospice staff encouraged us to continue talking to Mom, saying that she could still hear us. As each shift changed, the nurses and doctors repeated the same phrase, as they would stop at the doorway looking at Mom, "Wow! Look how peaceful she looks!" and "Her skin looks great!" My prayer had been answered: Momma was passing away peacefully.

Our brother Corey has been in jail for a couple of years now. I had to go through the respective channels to reach the chaplain to get news to Corey about Mom. I was able to speak with him and put him on speakerphone to talk to Mom. We each had alone time with Momma as she lay there. The hospice house was very serene. There was a patio outside of her room and a water fountain almost next to the patio. I found myself sitting out there quite often, meditating and praying for Mom. She began transitioning on Wednesday, and on Friday afternoon, I was sitting alone with her. I told her how much I loved her and assured her that her kids were with her and that she would be okay. I kissed her on her forehead and hugged her. A thought came to mind, so I told Momma, "When you go, check on Clint and if he's ready, take him with you." Clint had no quality of life. Medically, he was sustaining, but he was living on liquid or puréed food, mostly bedridden, and unable to communicate.

Saturday morning, as Karla and I were folding up the sheets and blankets from each of our pallets (Marcus had gone to work with Charles), Karla was reaching for her purse, which was on a shelf just above Mom's head. Karla got a whiff of an odor we couldn't explain. We checked to see if maybe Mom had soiled herself, but she hadn't. I then focused on Mom's carotid pulse and didn't feel one. I called the nurse to confirm. At about 8:15 a.m., Mom passed away, five days after I last spoke with her. My mind is always questioning the unknown. The day I went to Ruby Tuesday's, I donated $5 to charity. I sometimes wonder if smelling the lemons, then seeing the lemons, was a test. Had I donated the $20 bill that was in my wallet, would we have had 20 more days with Mom instead of five? Call me silly, it's just how my brain works sometimes. I suppose I won't understand the meaning of the lemons until the next time I see Momma. She will tell me.

Mom had asked to be buried at a reserved gravesite at her church in Georgia. On Sunday afternoon, on our way to Georgia, Marcus, Charles, and I decided to stop and check in on Clint since it was on the way. However, it was late in the day, and he was already sleeping. Marcus and I both kissed Clint, and when I went to hug him, I whispered in his ear, "Momma might be dropping by; if she does, it's okay if you want to go with her." The following day, Monday, in between making Mom's funeral arrangements, I had my monthly call with Clint's care team. Everything was status quo: no changes to medications or his care, and he was doing well. A few months prior, Clint had gone through an episode that prompted the doctor to discuss signing a DNR for him. After a long discussion, I knew it was time and signed the DNR.

We held Mom's funeral on Wednesday, one week after she began transitioning. It was a great ceremony, and her church family loved us, providing a feast of some of the best Southern cooking—all in keeping with a good down-home, Southern tradition of feeding the family of the deceased. Charles and I drove home, only to catch a flight to Kentucky the next day to spend time with our kids. Two days later, on Saturday, at approximately 8 a.m. (one week after Mom's passing, almost to the exact time), I got a call from Clint's nurse. "Julie! I don't know what's going on, but I think you and your family need to get here as soon as possible. There has been a significant shift in Clint, and I think he has begun the process of transitioning." I paused, took a breath, and sighed. "I know what's happening. Our momma passed away a week ago—she is there to get Clint." I told the nurse I was out of town and would not make it there in time but would call my other siblings, and they would be there.

Marcus drove over immediately, and Renée soon followed. Renée couldn't make it down in time to be with Momma when she passed away. She wasn't about to let her brother go without being by his side. They sat with Clint all night, Renée singing "Jesus Loves Me" to Clint and they both reading scriptures to him. Clint passed away a little after 2 p.m. on Sunday. The care he received from that VA home was incredible. Very compassionate and sincere care for their residents. His nurse cried when he passed, as I'm sure many nurses do when caring for someone for a long period of time. Clint was her "buddy," and he listened to (responded to) her the minute she would walk in the room; he would smile.

End of Chapter Takeaways

Own the fact that you are your loved one's voice. If they have not taken the steps to put in place their last will and testament, a power of attorney (there are different types), and a living will that identifies who they want to act as their medical surrogate, please take the initiative and schedule for them an appointment with a legal team or estate planning attorney immediately. Not everyone understands the importance of having this conversation, but it needs to happen sooner than later! Knowing your loved one's wishes truly takes weight off your shoulders and it acts like they handed you a road map to help you navigate the rough road ahead. There could be other legal documents that would benefit them. Speak with an attorney about what would be in their best interest to have in place.

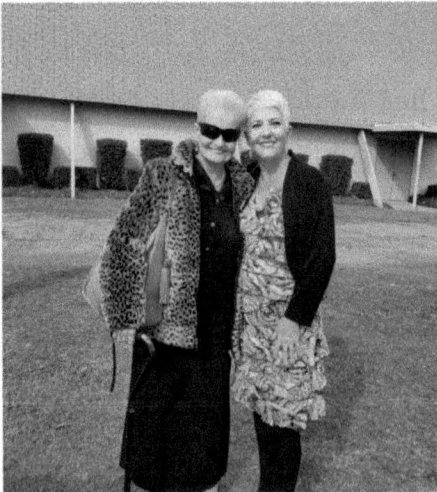

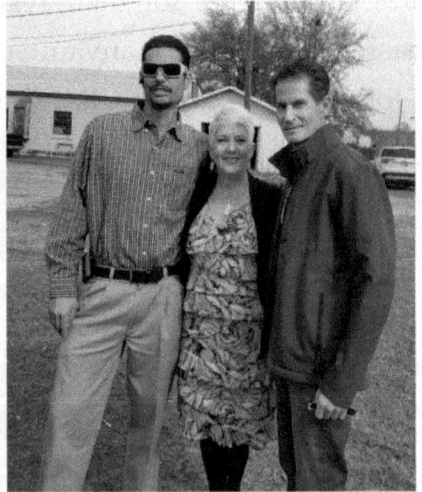

(left) Momma & Karla
(right) Corey, Karla, Clint, 2020

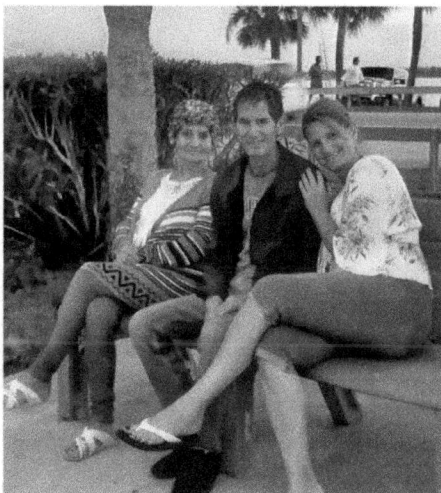

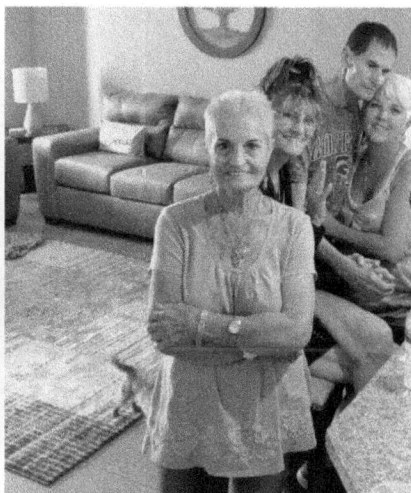

(left) Momma, Clint, Julie—move to Tampa
(right) Momma, Renee', Clint, & Karla—after
moving Mom into Tampa, 2020

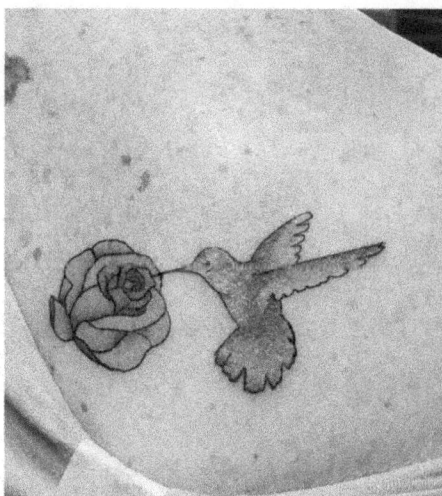

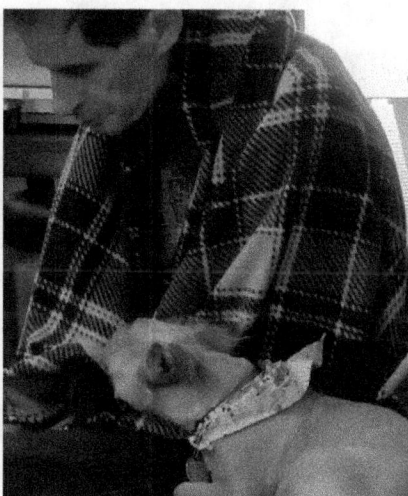

(left) Momma getting her first tattoo at age 81 *in* 2021
(right) Little Charlie comforting Clint prior
to moving to new apartment, 2020

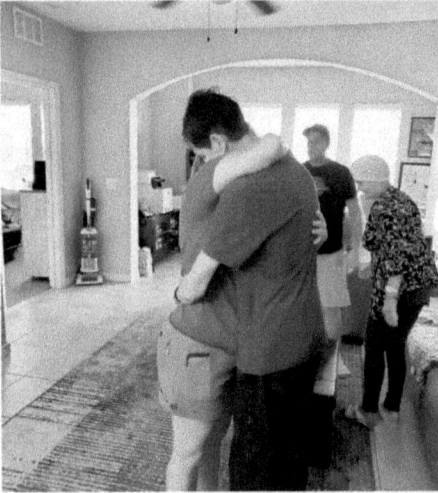

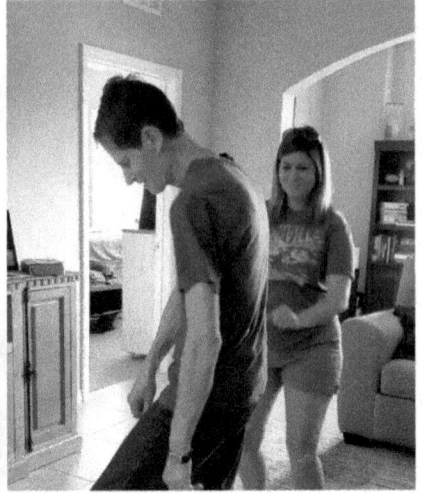

(left) Amy & Mike visiting Clint
(right) Clint & Amy Dancing, 2020

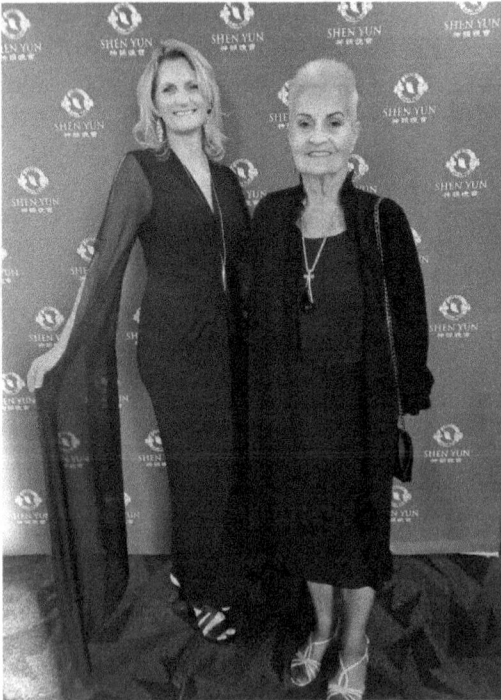

Julie & Mom attending
Shen Yun, 2022

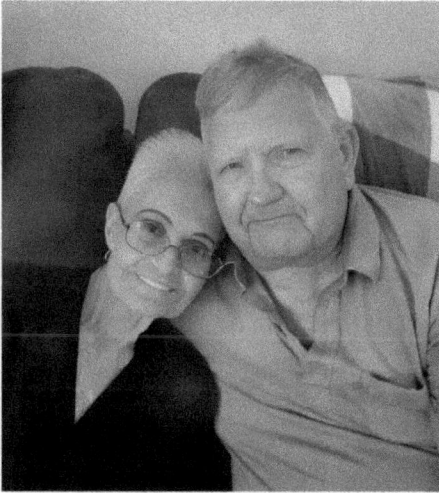

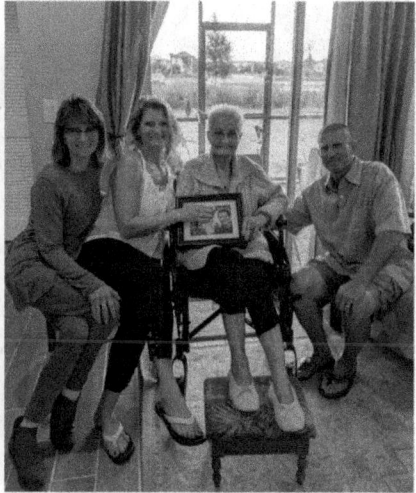

(left) Momma & Cousin-Tom, came to visit in 2022
(right) Thanksgiving in Jacksonville, 2021

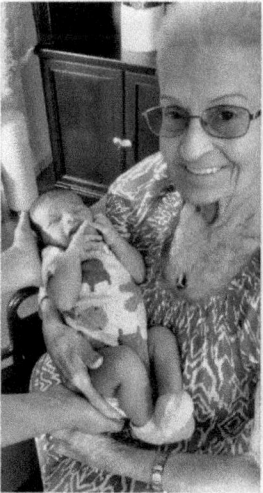

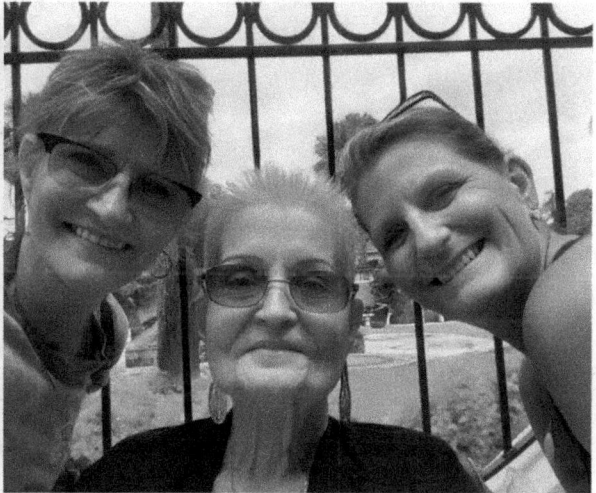

(left) Grandma-ma holding the youngest great-grandson
(right) Renee, Momma, Julie, 2022

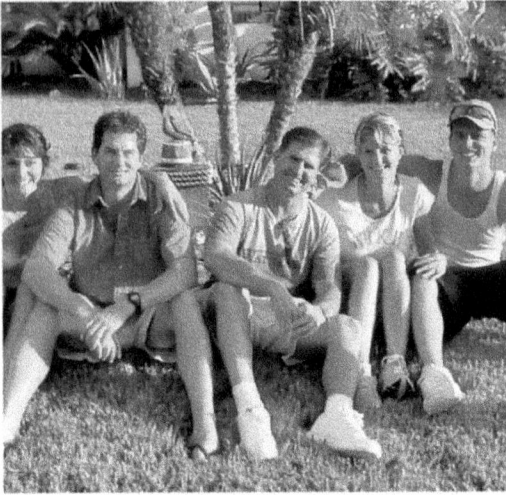

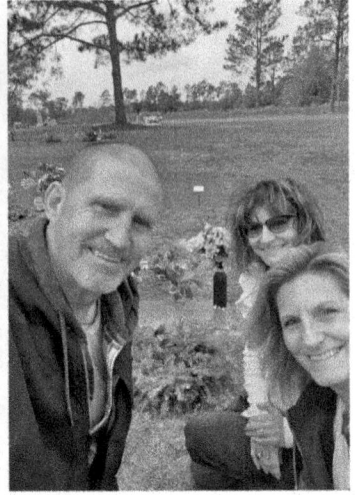

(left) Renee', Clint, Marcus, Julie, Corey
(Karla was gone that day) in 2010
(right) Marcus, Renee', & Julie at Daddy's Gravesite, 2024

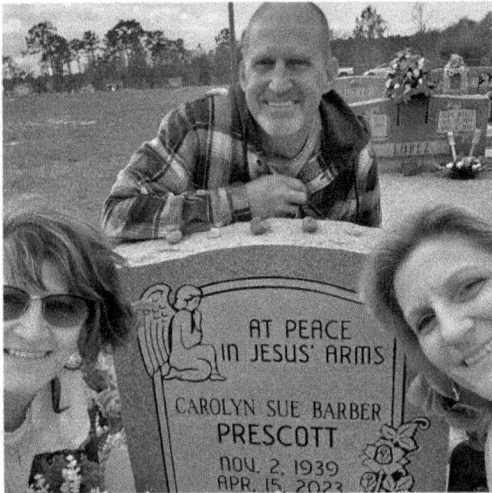

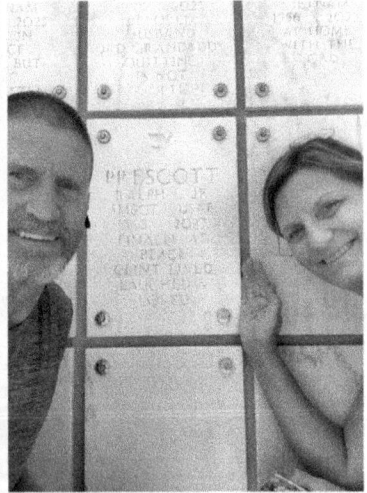

(left) Renee', Marcus & Julie at Momma's gravesite
(right) Marcus & Julie at Clint's gravesite in 2024

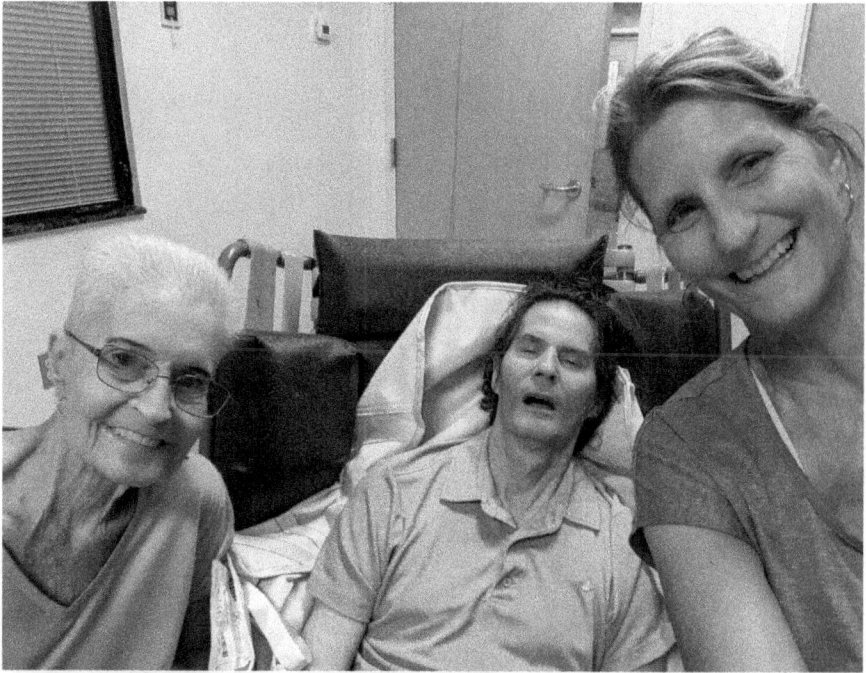

Momma, Clint, Julie - VA Home – 2022

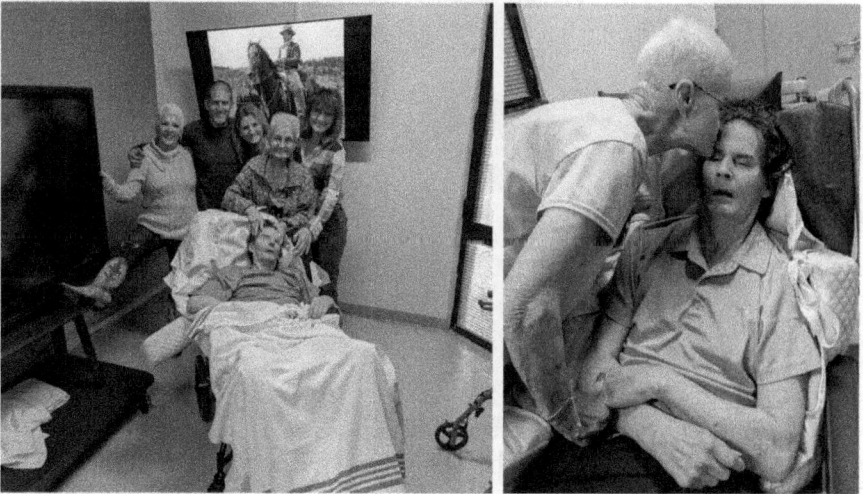

(left) Karla, Marcus, Julie, Momma, Renee', & Clint—VA Home
(right) Momma loving on her eldest, Clint - 2022

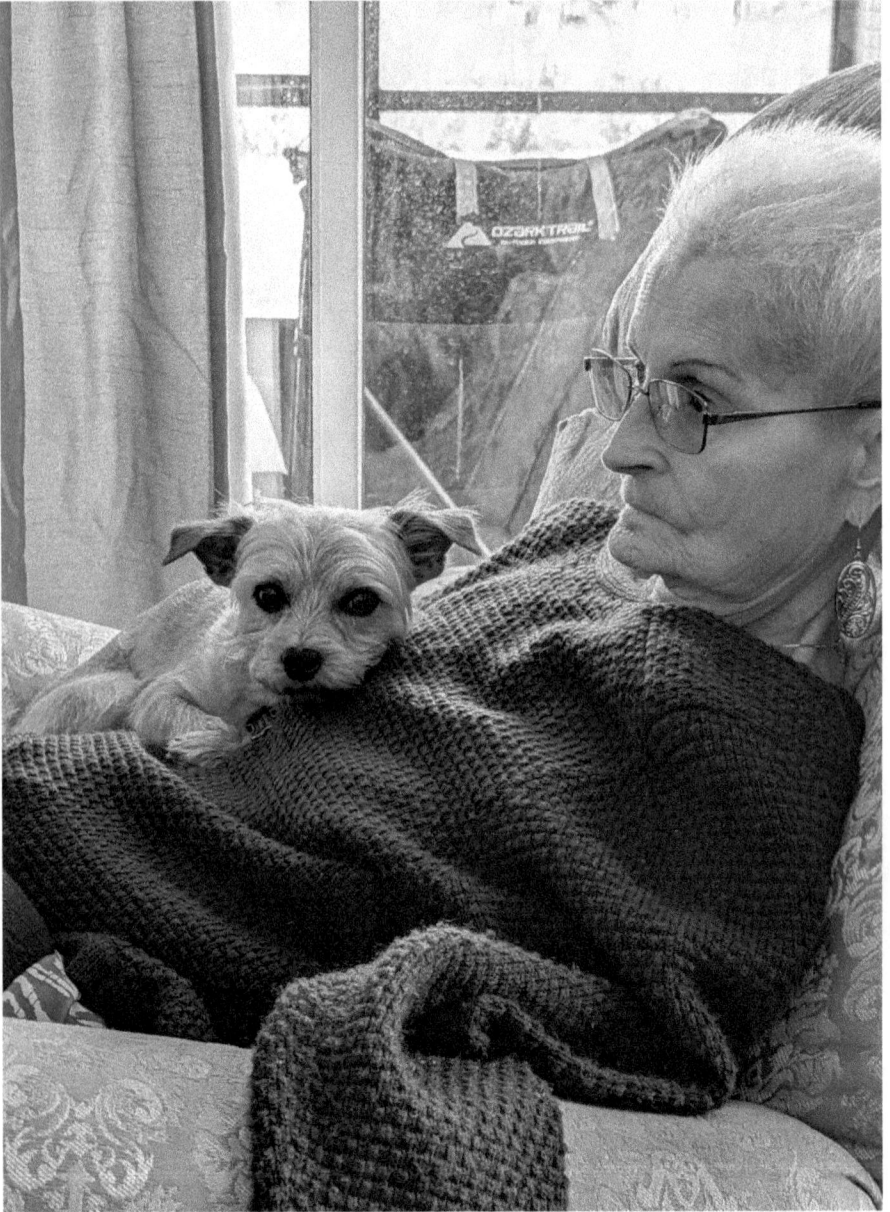
Figure 35 Charlie comforting Momma, 2021

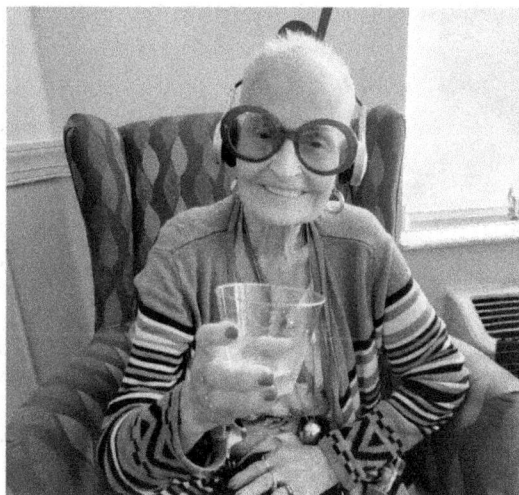

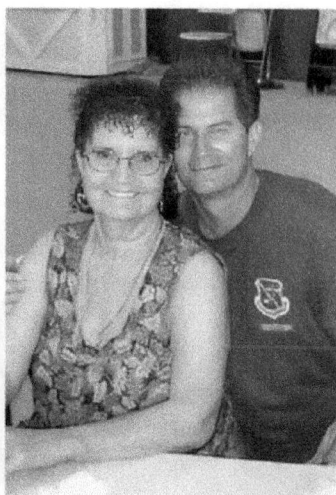

(left) Momma (10 days before passing) enjoying Disco Day at
the Senior Living Center in 2023
(right) Momma & Clint, together in life and death, 2008

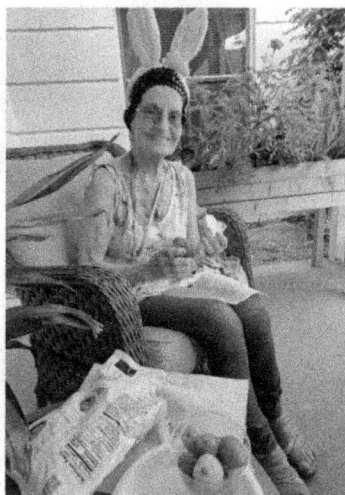

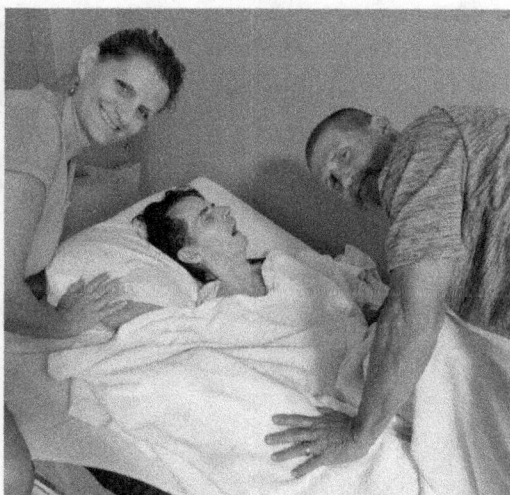

(left) Momma, Easter Sunday, 3 days before
slipping into transition in 2023
(right) Clint snoring logs, one week before he passed away

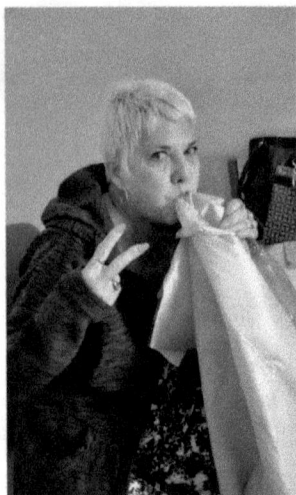

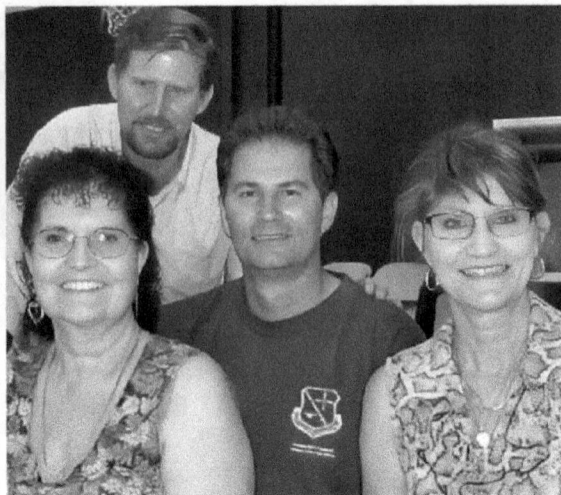

(left) Karla blowing up Marcus's bed at Hospice House, 2023
(right) Marcus, Momma, Clint, Renée in 2008

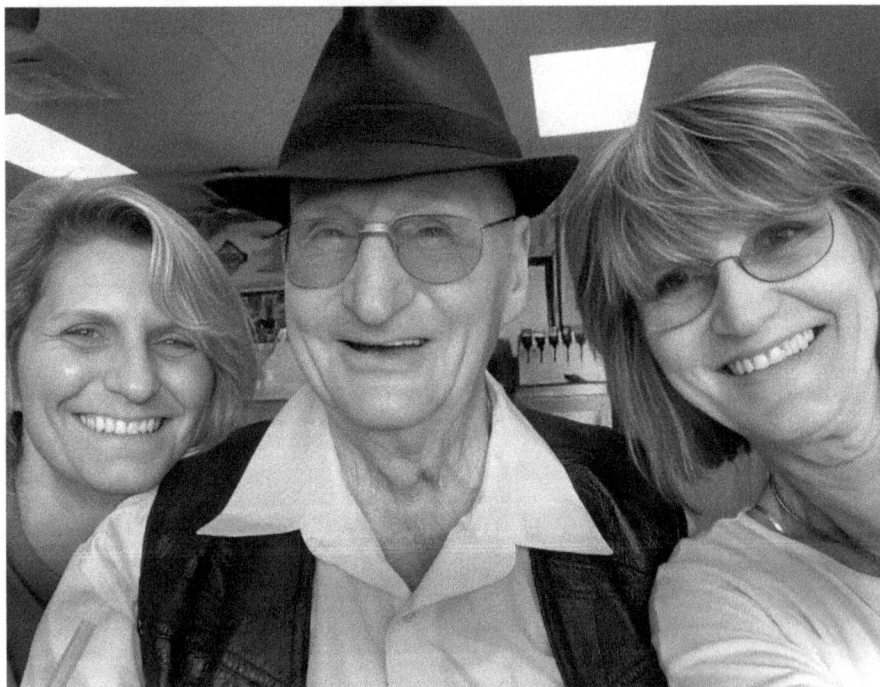

Julie, Daddy, Renée (daughter's surprise visit) 2019

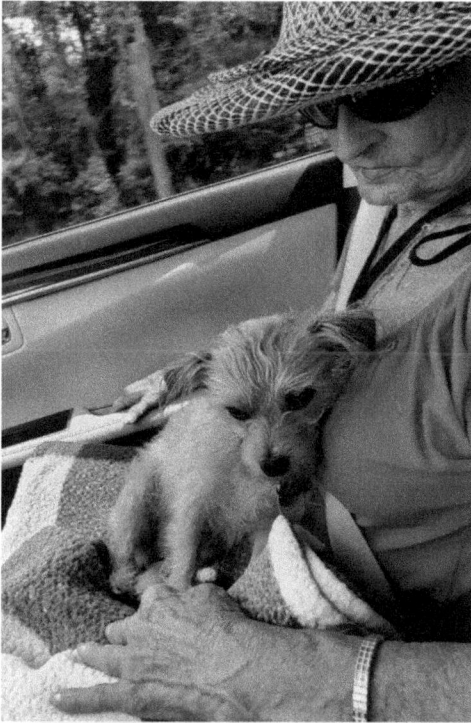

Charlie, happy to see Momma after a day at the spa, 2021

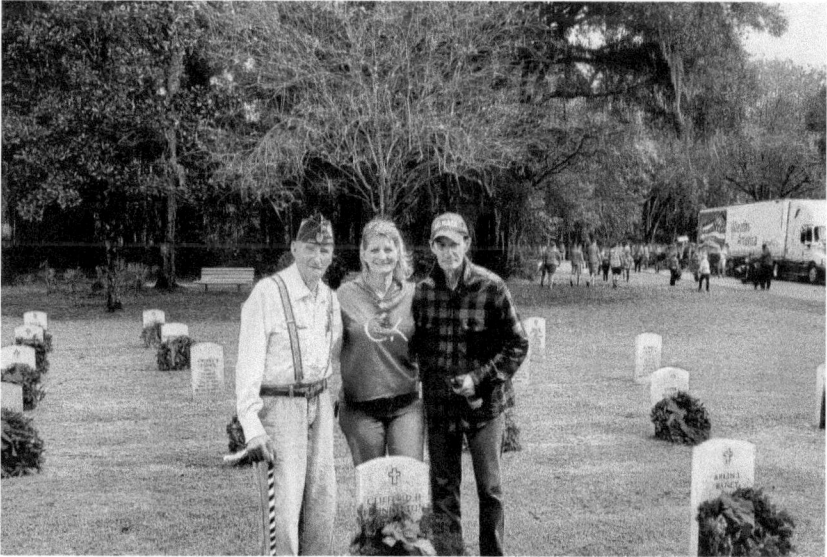

Daddy, Julie, Clint, Wreaths Across America in 2019

PART THREE

CLOSING CHAPTERS:
PUBLIC RESOURCES AND FINAL AFFAIRS

The expense of caring for the elderly or someone with a terminal disability has significantly increased in the last few decades. Study after study, news article after news article, is reporting the exponential rate of elderly care, especially for those with dementia.

In a 2023 AARP newsletter on political issues entitled "Valuing the Invaluable: 2023 Update Strengthening Supports for Family Caregivers," they state, *"In 2021, about 38 million family caregivers in the United States provided an estimated 36 billion hours of care to an adult with limitations in daily activities. The estimated economic value of their unpaid contributions was approximately $600 billion."* (https://www.aarp.org/content/dam/aarp/ppi/2023/3/valuing-the-invaluable-2023-update.doi.10.26419-2Fppi.00082.006.pdf). $600 billion! How do families survive?

I would surmise that many don't. The struggle is real. Fortunately, our government has programs in place to assist the elderly and disabled from assisting with your healthcare options, in-home care, or placement into a nursing home. All can be easily found on the internet; however, I will cover some of them in the following chapter. Unfortunately, some of the agencies have processes in place that make it difficult to get to an approval, and appealing those decisions is too often the "norm" and not the "exception."

The last chapter will cover the importance of having your estate planning documents in place. That could be as simple as a last will and testament and power of attorney, or as complex as a complete trust portfolio. Regardless, you and your loved ones need "something" written down that answers the question "What happens when... (fill in the blank)?"

CHAPTER FIVE
NAVIGATING SYSTEMS OF GOVERNMENT SUPPORT

W e've discussed the importance of having an emotional support system in place, such as family, friends, faith organizations, or even groups within the disease or disability community. But there are also systems the government has in place for those needing assistance.

Depending on your situation—financial, guidance, or both—the US government has programs in place to assist those in need. All of it can be confusing, but it doesn't have to be. I know that at first glance, when you hear about Medicare, Medicaid, the Veterans Administration, long-term care insurance, life insurance, and elder services, you may already have preconceived ideas about what each of them offers, but let's put those ideas on pause for a moment. You need to understand how each of these programs may offer exactly what you have been searching for.

I will start first with the more common understanding of each of these programs. Medicare is often thought of for those in their retirement years. But what is it? Medicare is health insurance that must be applied for when you reach the age of 65. You can apply earlier than 65 if you begin receiving Social Security retirement benefits as early as age 62. The Social Security Administration has put together a brief information packet that can answer many of your questions about what and when to apply for those benefits at this link:

https://www.ssa.gov/pubs/EN-05-10035.pdf

Regarding Medicare, there are two options to choose from: "Original Medicare" or "Medicare Advantage." Original Medicare has two parts: Part A, which covers your hospital stays, skilled nursing facility care, hospice care, and home health care, and Part B, which covers your doctors, outpatient and home health care, durable medical equipment (like a walker), and many preventive services like shots and yearly wellness visits. There is also a Medicare Advantage Plan (a.k.a. Part C), which has a higher premium and will include Parts A and B, but will also include Part D, which covers prescriptions, and most will also include a vision and dental plan. Medicare does a complete job explaining these options on their website at:

www.medicare.gov

When Momma moved in with me, she was already on a Medicare Advantage Plan, which was great because the prescriptions were included as well as the dental and vision plans. She wore dentures, and the set she had was the same one she received in the late 1970s. They were worn down and no longer sitting right due to her weight loss. Once she moved in with me, the process of switching her to a service plan in our area was relatively easy. Time-consuming, but again, the website does a great job at breaking down your options to help you pick which plan is best suited for your needs. The plan we went with also offered transportation. This came in very handy while Clint was still under my care. Although my church family was very supportive, there were times when no one was available to take Mom to a doctor's appointment. As a caregiver for two family members, it was easier to have the insurance transportation service take her to her appointment than trying to find someone to care for Clint (in the advanced stages of frontotemporal dementia) for a few hours. I will also share that I took it a step further by preparing a small binder for Mom, listing the time and location of her appointment and the name of the doctor she was seeing. In Tampa, she went to Moffitt Cancer Center for both chemotherapy and radiation therapy, and the facility is huge! I would get lost. So, to help Mom, I made sure everything was written out, including the number to call when she was ready to be picked up. It worked!

After we moved, however, that transportation service wasn't available on the new service plan. Thank goodness for Uber! I downloaded the app to Mom's phone and walked her through the process. At her age, technology was always a challenge. Thank goodness Uber already had implemented a process in their app where I could schedule her ride. At the end of the day, it was all about planning and thinking outside of the box.

Medicare has online access, and sooner rather than later, have them log in to their account and appoint an **authorized user**. This will be very important should—if your loved one becomes incompetent or incapacitated; then Medicare already identifies you as someone they are authorized to talk to about your loved one's benefits. You can learn more about assigning an authorized user here: https://www.medicare.gov/medicare-onlineforms/publicforms/cms10106.pdf

Medicare and Social Security often go hand in hand. If you apply for your Social Security benefits before age 65, Medicare will automatically enroll you for Parts A and B when you turn 65. For more information about Medicare, please visit this link:

https://www.medicare.gov/basics/get-started-with-medi-care/sign-up/when-does-medicare-coverage-start

Medicare is also available to those with disabilities under the age of 65. To receive it, you must first file for eligibility for a disability through Social Security. Social Security Disability Insurance (SSDI) is a benefit paid to those who "worked long enough and recently enough, paying Social Security taxes on your earnings." Then there is SSI (Supplemental Security Income), which provides monthly payments to adults and children with a disability or blindness who have income and resources below specific financial limits. Found at www.ssa.gov, SSI can also be paid to those over age 65 without disabilities that meet the financial qualifications. You can learn their process for applying and review their "strict definition of a disability" here:

https://www.ssa.gov/benefits/disability/qualify.html

We applied for SSDI for Clint. His initial application was denied immediately. We provided all his medical records, images, test results, and still he was denied. There is no sugar coating this process. It is time-consuming, frustrating, and sometimes arbitrary in what may be a very clear disability to you, but to them it is not. Inevitably, your initial application will get denied. You must remain persistent! Appeal! Appeal! Appeal! It sucks, and you feel it is a waste of your time as a caregiver. I agree with you! Fight it anyway.

Once approved, SSA will backdate your approval to the date of your initial application. To review SSA's Checklist for Online Adult Disability Application, visit:

https://www-origin.ssa.gov/hlp/radr/10/ovw001-check-list.pdf

Spend some time on this website, researching "How You Qualify" and "What We Mean by Disability." To not only play the game but to stay in it, you need to learn the rules—their rules—and play accordingly. In preparation of this topic, I discovered "Quick Disability Determinations" on the SSA website. Learn more about it here:

https://www.ssa.gov/disabilityresearch/qdd.htm?ab=3

Next is Medicaid www.medicaid.gov. Some of you may be familiar with Medicaid, based on your income and/or inability to obtain health insurance. That is one side of Medicaid. Here, I want to focus on obtaining Medicaid benefits for the purpose of seeking long-term healthcare for someone who is elderly, or anyone with disabilities who cannot afford their healthcare needs at home or needs to be placed into a facility to receive the care they need. Often confused with Medicare, it has included the following description of the difference between the two on its website: Medicare *is federal health insurance for anyone age 65 and older, and some people under 65 with certain disabilities or conditions.* **Medicaid** *is a joint federal and state program that provides health coverage for some people with limited income and resources. Medicaid offers* *benefits like nursing home care, personal care services, and assistance paying for Medicare premiums and other costs.* When it comes to long-term care facilities, each state has its own process to follow when applying. In the state of Florida, they have Elder Affairs-Florida www.elderaffairs.org.

Now, if you are proactive like me and try to begin the application process for Medicaid to cover the cost of long-term care facilities ahead of moving your loved one, you need to pump your brakes. As I learned the hard way, although it made sense to initiate the Medicaid approval process in preparation for moving my brother into a facility, I wanted the comfort of knowing that the bill would be covered and there would be no financial stress. Unfortunately, all I did was create confusion for those processing my application. When a Medicaid processor would call me for additional information, they kept asking, "Which facility is your brother in?" To which I would reply, "None yet. I am waiting for approval from you?!"

I had explored applying for Medicaid to get government assistance should the time come, and I "had" to place Clint in a home. Every state has an Elder Care office (Department of Elder Affairs) to seek assistance for the elderly, for example, medical care, housing, or to report elderly abuse. I didn't know what I didn't know. I thought I could simply apply for Medicaid and get Clint approved "in case" he needed it. I consider myself a proactive person and self-reliant. I can read and am able to follow directions well, so I went to the Medicaid website and began the process of getting Clint approved. I then reached out to Elder Affairs (even though he was not considered "elder" by age, he was a disabled adult and eligible for assistance), only to discover that I put the cart before the horse. Being the process person that I am, my expectation is that organizations in the business of serving the community will have clearly mapped out process steps for anyone to follow. That includes incorporating any other agency that is a part of their process. I expect an "easy" button. Sad to say, when dealing with government agencies, the "easy" button doesn't exist. At least, not yet.

Medicaid's process is for you to first place your loved one into a facility. While you are still trying to figure out a way to pay the bill, have the social worker at the facility assist you in applying for assistance. Did you catch that? My Southern, somewhat country-girl mind kicked in and said, "Well, that's *bassackwards!*" (*a.k.a. ass-backwards*). "What? -the-What!" And you wonder why government programs are so complicated. They really don't have to be. Nonetheless, the bottom line is you cannot initiate a Medicaid application for long-term care until you have already placed your loved one in a long-term care facility. You will need to be prepared financially to pay for at least the first full month (possibly two or three months), to include any application fees and/or deposits to the facility your loved one lives in.

Another "need-to-know" about applying for Medicaid is understanding their eligibility requirements and their very invasive methods of determining your approval. You should also know about the required "payback" of funds paid by them to cover your loved one's care. I'll restate that last part: once approved by Medicaid, there will be a debt that must be repaid for those who are 55 years and older. "According to federal and state law, the money that the Florida Medicaid program pays on behalf of a Medicaid recipient is a debt owed back to the state. Upon the death of the Medicaid recipient, the Medicaid program files a claim against the decedent's estate in order to seek reimbursement for the amount owed." https://bit.ly/41UrwW5

That topic isn't addressed while you are applying for assistance. People are often blindsided with this information while they are dealing with the loss of their loved one and trying to focus on planning their funeral and managing what's left of their estate. For more information about Florida's Statewide Medicaid Managed Care Long-Term Care program, please visit the LTC website at:

http://ahca.myflorida.com/Medi-caid/statewide_mc/smmc_ltc.shtml.

Once I understood their process and after reviewing the eligibility requirements, we discovered that our brother was not eligible for Medicaid due to his receiving his military retirement and SSDI from Social Security. This may sound like enough money, but it wasn't, because of the level of care that Clint required. According to assisted living facilities that have memory care units, we were ultimately told he needed a skilled nursing facility where all his activities of daily living were done for him, plus the administration of medications. We were looking at a minimum of $12,000 per month. NO ONE in our family could afford to pay that bill. The physical, mental, and emotional demands already placed on myself, and my mom had become more than we could bear. Clint needed 24-hour care, and I was exhausted. I did apply for him to be placed into one of the many

VA nursing homes in Florida; however, they have their own convoluted process that required me to send in updated bank statements and doctors' progress notes every two to three months. Time and again we were told that his application was rejected due to the potential for him to be combative and he did not have a service-connected disability, which moved him to the bottom of the list to have his application reviewed. It wasn't until I was at my wits' end that I took Clint to a VA emergency room one night to have him evaluated for severe constipation. I did get assistance with placement into a different VA nursing home than the one I applied to. While speaking with the doctor and eventually a social worker, I explained Clint's need to be placed. They began working with me to not only allow him to be admitted to the VA hospital for medical care for the constipation but then continued to care for him until they helped me find a VA facility to take over his care.

If your loved one is a veteran, reach out to a Veteran Service Officer (VSO) in your county. They can assist you with navigating the VA system and applying for or submitting a disability claim to include updating an existing disability rating. You will need your loved one's DD Form 214. All branches receive a DD Form 214 when they leave the military. This is their proof of being in the military. Regardless of whether your loved one was active duty or in the National Guard or Reserves, a VSO can assist you. You can also visit www.va.gov and find more information about locating a VA clinic or hospital in your area to take your military veteran in for healthcare.

We often hear horror stories that happen in "nursing homes," and it is these stories that left such a negative impression on our family. None of us wanted any of our family members to be placed in a nursing home, not to mention the expense of being in one. This is why Mom chose to move Grams into her home when Grams could no longer live on her own with Alzheimer's. It is why Mom agreed to help care for her daughter-in-law after her Alzheimer's diagnosis and why Mom also moved Clint in with her. Mom "knew" she would provide better—and less expensive—care for her loved ones, until it became too much.

I continued that practice when I moved Clint and Momma in with me. The fear of strangers caring for my brother and not doing things the way I know he prefers, plus the expense of everything, were strong motivating factors. We were not a family of means. Even if we wanted our family members to go into a home, we couldn't afford it. I was recently reminded of adults who do not have any siblings and the stress of caring for their aging parents. Can you imagine being an only child and having to manage your parents' care when they can no longer do it themselves? Maybe that's you, now. Although I am not an only child, I do empathize with your challenges and want you to know that there is light at the end of the tunnel. Hang on! Stay strong! Seek therapy, join a gym, go for a walk, seek out nursing homes in your area that offer respite care. Just know that "This too, shall pass!"

When I don't understand something, I quickly find myself jumping down rabbit holes to aid my learning. Some rabbit holes are unnecessary, and time wasted, but all in all, it is still research.

Just as Edison found 1,000 ways not to make the light bulb, the time I spent learning and navigating the systems in place for the elderly and disabled served a purpose. For example, in my research, I discovered there are many types of elderly care: senior living facilities, assisted living facilities, memory care units, nursing homes, skilled nursing facilities, and rehabilitation facilities. They all allow residency based on a "functional assessment" test. A functional assessment tests the different levels of activities of daily living (ADLs) that a resident can do on their own. It was this type of test that told me the level of care that Clint needed, in the advanced stages of frontotemporal dementia.

Some of these facilities offer housing based on the progression of the residents' disease. For example, if your loved one is still able to do all of their ADLs, is still very active and able to go shopping on their own but can no longer drive, moving them into a senior living facility allows them to live on their own and participate in daily activities. As they age, they may get to a point where they aren't as active and maybe need help managing their medications. They can move from the senior living wing to the assisted living wing of the facility. If dementia sets in and they begin to decline in their ADLs, they can then be moved to the memory care wing of the facility.

A skilled nursing facility is for those patients who cannot do any of their ADLs and require 24 hours of nursing care. I didn't understand all these differences while Clint was under my care, and I was trying to decide when I needed to move him to a facility. Trying to absorb all this new information while also caring for a loved one can be challenging and confusing. Learning the level of care that Clint required and the cost that came with that care became very discouraging.

If your loved one has life insurance and/or long-term care insurance, be sure to review it and ensure that the premiums are paid and that you know all there is to know about what the policy offers. There may be certain restrictions when it comes to payouts upon death or when placing them into a facility. Also, have your loved one review their beneficiaries list. Make sure it reflects your loved one's wishes and that the beneficiaries' contact information is up to date. I'll cover more about having certain end-of-life documents in place in the next chapter.

When your loved one serves in the military, they could possibly be eligible for various benefits through the Veterans Administration (VA). Not only does this include medical care, but also assistance with burials and memorials. I recommend you start by locating the Veteran Service Officer (VSO) in your county to determine which benefits they are eligible for. You will need a copy of your loved one's DD Form 214, if they were ever in the military. A VSO will let you know of any other documents needed. You can also go directly to a VA clinic or hospital and speak with their admissions office. There you will find a DVA (Department of Veterans Affairs) officer. Like a VSO, they can assist you in determining your loved one's eligibility status.

Here are some links to assist you in your search:

- Find VA locations: https://www.va.gov/find-locations/
- Get copies of medical records: https://www.va.gov/health-care/get-medical-records/
- Find VA specific forms: https://www.va.gov/find-forms/

- Find resources (e.g., burials and memorials): https://www.va.gov/resources/
- Find outreach services & events: https://www.va.gov/outreach-and-events/events/

End of Chapter Takeaways

I believe the key takeaway here is to educate yourself in all that is available to your loved one. From federal to state, there are programs in place that can assist you with medical care and/or funding, and insurance plans that offer benefits they will need. The systems in place are established for those in need. Educate yourself and take advantage of all that is offered and available. It just might be the saving grace you are hoping for.

CHAPTER SIX
PREPARING FOR END OF LIFE

What Happens to My Family and My Belongings When I Die?
That is a great question to ask. It is never too early to ask yourself hard questions like this. Estate planning is something that everyone, not just the rich, must do. Death is inevitable. We are ALL going to die one day. We all need to be thinking about what is going to happen to all this "stuff" in my home. The first step, though, is taking inventory of all you have.

Being in the military, moving from one assignment to the next every 3–5 years, we quickly learned about the bad habits of collecting "stuff" we didn't need or even use. You can ask any veteran who has had to move multiple times about the number of boxes they had left unopened from a previous move, and I would venture to say that 90% would say "A LOT!"

Each time we moved, we would find boxes packed up from the previous house that were never reopened. So, we began asking the first hard question: "Do we really need it?" If the "stuff" has stayed in a box for over three years, do we really need it? We would try to weed out items annually, if not during packing for the next move. If an item (or box) fell into the category of unused, we would immediately make the decision to either give it away to someone who needed it, donate it to organizations like Goodwill or the Breast Cancer Society, or dispose of it if it could not be repurposed for something else.

As painful as it may sound to go through a garage or attic full of unused stuff, consider the plight it may put your family through when *they* must go through it all themselves after you have passed away. As a caregiver, I had to help my mom go through this very painful process of deciding what to keep or give away—to give it to this daughter or give it to that grandson. I wanted to avoid asking my mom to sit with me as I went through her boxes, but I knew it was best if I presented it to her gently and asked her to tell me what she wanted to do with everything.

Momma had a lot of "stuff." She still has a lot of stuff that was left behind in her trailer that our youngest brother must now go through. I shared with Momma that I knew how important her things were to her, and I wanted to make sure that I knew who *she* wanted to have them. Momma didn't like to talk about death; most people don't. It forces you to face the truth of your inevitability, and when you aren't ready to go, ignoring it allows you to pretend that you will live forever. It took a few days, if not weeks, but eventually, with me helping Mom go through her boxes, we were able to donate a lot to Goodwill, local churches, and label specific items to be left to her children and grandchildren. Some of those items were given to them before Momma passed away, which helped her to know that the right person received her gift.

What happens to your family when you pass? They will be sad, of course. However, knowing your wishes and desires will ease their sadness, aid in the healing after losing you, and prepare their lives for moving forward. Hopefully, it can also ease any conflict between family members, knowing that all you left behind will be distributed according to your wishes. Even when our dad passed away, he called each of us to tell us where he left his will and that the few items he possessed were all kept in a shed. Renée went up a couple of weekends before he passed away to spend time with Daddy so he could show her where everything was, and she began going through his belongings. He wanted to make sure we each received what he wanted us to have.

Now, Daddy and Clint had a last will and testament, while Mom had a trust in place. What's the difference? A last will and testament is a single legal document that lists what you want done with all that belongs to you after you pass away, including all your assets and property. It also allows you to identify one person as an executor to execute your wishes according to your will. A trust is another legal document that allows you to transfer your assets to a trustee to manage before and after you pass, then distribute them to your beneficiaries according to your will. Yes, a Trust can become effective before you pass, while a will does not become effective until after you pass away.

Knowing your loved one's wishes for the level or extent of care will also help in organizing their support group. For me, our family was the first line of defense. Because we recognized early on to document our mother and brother's wishes for when they died, we all knew not only what to do with their assets, but how they wanted to be cared for should the day come that we could no longer manage it, and how they wanted to leave this world.

We ensured both Mom and Clint had their last will and testament, power of attorney, and advanced healthcare directive before it became too late for either of them to legally sign these documents. Hopefully, you are close enough to know your loved one's desires or dreams, as well as their wishes regarding their health.

I strongly recommend and encourage you to get these documents in place now, even if you or your loved ones are not showing any signs of disease. You never know what a day holds; you could get into a car accident, leaving you unconscious and unable to communicate your needs or wishes. Estate planning is not just for the rich, nor is it just for your "estate." Seek counsel sooner than later. I've listed some resources at the end of this book.

There is also a question of having to go through probate court. Probate is a legal process that distributes a deceased person's assets, appoints executors, and validates wills. When you have a trust in place, the process of transferring assets has technically already taken place; therefore, the court only validates the trust and allows that process to proceed. With only a will, the probate court must still validate the will and officially recognize the executor named in it to begin distributing assets accordingly. When there is no will in place, the estate must still go through probate and the court will distribute the estate according to the order of succession in the state's intestate laws (intestate means when someone passes away without a will in place). This could be a very long process and an expensive one, as your beneficiaries are expected to pay all court costs.

You shouldn't wait until you're on your deathbed to consider having a last will and testament or power of attorney in place. When your children turn 18, you should consider having them sign a power of attorney in the event something happens to them, causing them to become unconscious or incapacitated, because they are legally adults, and you can no longer say, "Well, I'm the mother!" They are adults and, as such, have a say in what's best for them. Since I am not an attorney, I must give this disclaimer and recommend you speak to an estate planning attorney or even an online legal team (with attorneys on staff).

Based on my own experience, our family made sure both Mom and Clint had the following legal documents in place before they reached a point of being medically diagnosed as incompetent: last will and testament, durable power of attorney, living will, and advanced medical directive (naming a medical surrogate).

There are different types of powers of attorney (POA): medical, financial, and durable. Each carries different, if not limited, powers. Speak with your legal team about the differences and which is the most relevant one for you to have. One important thing to understand about a POA is that it ceases to exist upon the death of the person (known as the "principal") it comes from. Whatever access you may be granted as a POA while they are alive will stop when they die. Therefore, you need to consider other alternatives to manage whatever you're managing as a POA once they pass away. This is another important difference between having the power of attorney in place and having a trust in place that names a trustee to manage assets. In a trust, a trustee is appointed to continue managing assets after death.

If you have chosen not to have a trust in place, the next best thing to discuss with your legal team and your loved one (if their mental capacity isn't an issue) is for the named POA to be added to all financial accounts and property deeds —meaning adding the POA as an account holder or co-owner on a property deed.

For example, let's say your mother has a terminal illness and assigns you as her financial power of attorney to manage her bills, allowing you access to her checking account. As a POA, you have the right to write checks to pay her bills, but when she passes away, that access will end. The bank will freeze her checking account in anticipation of the executor of her will or trustee (if applicable) to distribute her assets accordingly (a checking account is considered an asset). Keeping this example in mind, when you become the POA and your mother agrees, have her add you to her accounts. This will allow your efforts to continue to manage her estate without any interruptions or delays from the processes of probate court. **You should also check with the bank to learn their process for when an account owner passes away.** This will aid in your preparation and decision-making.

You can seek out estate planning attorneys in your area. You can also find online legal teams such as LegalShield or Rocket Lawyer. If your family does not have a lot of assets and you are comfortable with putting something simple together, office supply stores like Staples or Office Depot sell generic, fill-in-the-blank last will and testament and power of attorney forms.

Finally, at the very least, your loved one can handwrite their last will and testament (known as a holographic will) and have two uninterested parties (not family) sign as witnesses. In the state of Florida, a last will and testament does not have to be notarized, but it may be in your best interest to have it notarized, where the two witnesses can be identified by a notary and their signatures notarized on what's known as a self-proving affidavit. Ask your notary more about this document.

Once your loved one has these legal documents in place, I recommend digitally storing them in a safe and secure place like My Life & Wishes Legacy Vault. This allows whomever your loved one has appointed to access and locate these documents 24/7 from the comfort of their own home, especially when they live in other states or even another country. The founder, Jon Braddock, and his wife, Michelle, found themselves in a tough spot when her parents passed away. Not knowing their wishes and desires, then struggling to locate documents for when it came time to manage and distribute their estate, created more challenges than they were expecting. Jon wrote a book called *Click Here When I Die!* I recommend you read it. You can learn more about My Life & Wishes here: www.iamtheirvoice.com

End of Chapter Takeaways

We all want to live a long time. We want to keep having fun with our families, our children, our friends. The takeaway from this chapter is acknowledging and accepting that our days on this Earth are numbered. Unfortunately, we don't always know when our time will be but know that it will come. Having a conversation about what-ifs for when your loved one—and even yourself—will pass away is needed sooner rather than later. Think of it as giving a road map to your family. Having estate planning documents, like a last will and testament, power of attorney, or even a trust in place, will serve as a guide to those left behind to locate and distribute your possessions as you would want them to be given. These documents also serve as guides for whomever ends up as your caregiver, should you become mentally incapacitated. Trust that the sooner you have these legal documents in place, the sooner you can get back to enjoying every day with those you love and doing the activities you love to do. You will walk a little lighter, knowing that if something were to happen to you overnight, you've done your part—or your loved one did theirs—and will be at peace no matter what the day may bring.

REFERENCES

AARP. Valuing the Invaluable: 2023 Update Strengthening Supports for Family Caregivers. https://www.aarp.org/content/dam/aarp/ppi/2023/3/valuing-the-invaluable-2023-update.doi.10.26419-2Fppi.00082.006.pdf

Alzheimer's Organization. www.alz.org

Association of Frontotemporal Degeneration. https://www.theaftd.org/

Association of Frontotemporal Degeneration. Overview of Frontotemporal Degeneration. https://www.theaftd.org/what-is-ftd/disease-overview

The World Health Organization. "Key Facts" of worldwide dementia cases, https://www.who.int/news-room/fact-sheets/detail/dementia

Junger, Sebastian. *Tribe* (audio version). Hachette Audio. May 24, 2016.

Sandberg, Sheryl. *Lean In* (audio version). Random House Audio. Mar 11, 2013.

Sinek, Simon. *Leaders Eat Last* (audio version). Brillance Audio. Jan 7, 2014.

The Mayo Clinic. Understanding Sundowners. https://www.mayoclinic.org/diseases-conditions/alzheimers-disease/expert-answers/sundowning/faq-20058511#:~:text=The%20term%20%22sundowning%22%20refers%20to,Sundowning%20isn't%20a%20disease

Association of Frontotemporal Degeneration. Music Therapy for People with Dementia. https://www.the-aftd.org/posts/1ftd-in-the-news/bbc-music-therapy-people-with-dementia/

Schneck, Corey. Stress and Anxiety Relief. Harmony and Healing: The Impact of Classical Music on Mental Health. https://www.piano-composer-teacher-london.co.uk/post/classical-music-and-mental-health

Newswire. The Science Behind Why Classical Music Is Good for Mental Health. https://myscena.org/newswire/the-science-behind-why-classical-music-is-good-for-mental-health/

Lottoland. The 8 Surprising Ways Music is Good for Your Health. https://www.lottoland.co.za/magazine/the-8-surprising-ways-rock-music-is-good-for-your-health.html

AARP. Nursing Home Dumping. April 19, 2021. https://www.aarp.org/caregiving/financial-legal/info-2021/nursing-home-dumping-lawsuit.html

Chapman, Gary. *The Five Love Languages*. Northfield Publishing. Chicago, IL. 2004.

Community Health at Johns Hopkins Bayview. Social Support Systems. Called to Care. https://www.hopkinsmedicine.org/about/community-health/johns-hopkins-bayview/services/called-to-care/social-support-systems

The American Cancer Society. www.cancer.org

Psychology Today. How To Manage Expectations. https://www.psychologytoday.com/us/blog/the-wisdom-of-anger/202309/how-to-manage-expectations

Stamets, Paul. Mushrooms as Medicine. NextMed Health. https://youtu.be/7agK0nkiZpA?si=9rvHsclucT2rAdhE

Chemotherapy and Radiation Side Effects, https://www.cancer.gov/about-cancer/treatment/side-effects/mouth-throat

Social Security Administration. www.ssa.gov

Social Security Administration Disability. https://www.ssa.gov/benefits/disability/qualify.html

Social Security Administration Information Packet. https://www.ssa.gov/pubs/EN-05-10035.pdf

Medicare. www.medicare.gov

Understanding When Medicare Starts. https://www.medicare.gov/basics/get-started-with-medicare/sign-up/when-does-medicare-coverage-start

Social Security Administration Online Adult Disability Application. https://www-origin.ssa.gov/hlp/radr/10/ovw001-checklist.pdf

Social Security Administration Quick Disability Determinations. https://www.ssa.gov/disabilityresearch/qdd.htm?ab=3

Medicaid. www.medicaid.gov

Elder Affairs-Florida. www.ederaffairs.org

Florida Medicaid Debt Payment. https://www.flmedicaidtplrecovery.com/flmedicaidtplrecovery.com/faqs/estate/index.html#:~:text=According%20to%20federal%20and%20state,reimbursement%20for%20the%20amount%20owed

Florida Statewide Medicaid Managed Care Long-Term Care Program. http://ahca.myflorida.com/Medicaid/statewide_mc/smmc_ltc.shtml

Florida Agency for Health Care Administration. http://ahca.myflorida.com

The Veterans Administration. www.va.gov

Authorized User Form for Medicare. https://www.medicare.gov/medicareonlineforms/publicforms/cms10106.pdf

VA locations. https://www.va.gov/find-locations/

Military Medical records. https://www.va.gov/healthcare/get-medical-records/

VA specific forms. https://www.va.gov/find-forms/

VA Resources (i.e., burials and memorials). https://www.va.gov/resources/

VA Outreach services & Events. https://www.va.gov/outreach-and-events/events/

Legal Shield. https://www.legalshield.com/

Rocket Lawyer. https://www.rocketlawyer.com/

My Life & Wishes Legacy Vault. www.swflnotaryclosings.com/legacy-vault

Teepa Snow. Positive Approach to Care. https://teepasnow.com/

Teepa Snow. YouTube Channel. https://www.youtube.com/channel/UCSXrEX7LkWOmfTaV6u1C7wQ

Teepa's GEMS Brain Change Model. https://youtu.be/Z6UVjp_y8HY?si=XG6FVB4MmSct9Gi2

Stepping Into Dementia's Reality: Advice From Teepa Snow | Brain Talks | Being Patient. https://youtu.be/EOCZInnLQd0?si=ec062Z-bwspRk9Vl

Time with Teepa. How Can We De-escalate Someone That is Agitated? https://www.youtube.com/watch?v=2kMjA5z8XAg

National Institute on Aging. https://www.nia.nih.gov/health/long-term-care/what-long-term-care

All About Birds. https://www.allaboutbirds.org/guide/Northern_Cardinal/id#:~:text=Male%20cardinals%20are%20brilliant%20red,wings%2C%20tail%2C%20and%20crest

CanCare. Cancer Support Groups Near You. https://www.cancare.org/

A Place for Mom. Finding Respite Care. https://www.aplaceformom.com/lp/respite-care

Free Downloads (Florida documents). https://longterm-caresolutionsllc.com/advancedirectives/

EPILOGUE

Another Valuable Resource

Another resource I found immensely valuable while caring for someone with dementia is an occupational therapist named Teepa Snow. You need only type her name into Google or, especially, YouTube to learn who this incredible person is and the value she brings to the dementia community. Teepa developed a system for caring for people with dementia that no other agency or entity has done. Her system is called Positive Approach to Care (PAC). I believe I was on the right track while caring for Clint because, before I found Teepa's teachings, I was practicing some of them. Seeing her PAC system gave me confidence in my caregiving and taught me many, many more things about how to best care for Clint. After moving Clint into an assisted living facility, I asked the staff if they were familiar with Teepa's teachings, and many had taken her courses. Knowing this added to my frustration because they weren't practicing them. I strongly encourage you to watch her videos. She incorporates a lot of role-plays to help you fully understand and immerse yourself in a situation. Here are a few to get you started.

1. Teepa's GEMS Brain Change Model: https://youtu.be/Z6UVjp_y8HY?si=XG6FVB4MmSct9Gi2
2. Stepping Into Dementia's Reality: Advice From Teepa Snow | Brain Talks | Being Patient: https://youtu.be/EOCZInnLQd0?si=ec062Z-bwspRk9Vl
3. Time with Teepa: How Can We De-escalate Someone That Is Agitated? https://www.youtube.com/watch?v=2kMjA5z8XAg

When you learn Teepa's GEMS and then think about my journey with Clint, you will realize each of his GEM moments as I experienced them.

Journal Entries (Dreams and Visits from Cardinals)
March 17, 2024

I was going through the pictures on my phone, and I came across one I had taken from my backyard on May 1, 2023, a few weeks after Mom and Clint's passing, and completely forgot about it. When I zoomed in, I realized that there were two cardinals. When I researched "Are all cardinals red?" this is what I found:

"Male cardinals are brilliant red all over, with a reddish bill and black face immediately around the bill. Females are pale brown overall with warm reddish tinges in the wings, tail, and crest. They have the same black face and red-orange bill." https://www.allaboutbirds.org/guide/Northern_Cardinal/id#:~:text=Male%20cardinals%20are%20brilliant%20red,wings%2C%20tail%2C%20and%20crest

Oh, my, goodness! That was Mom and Clint! Sitting on the roof of our condos, looking over the backyard where the pool is.

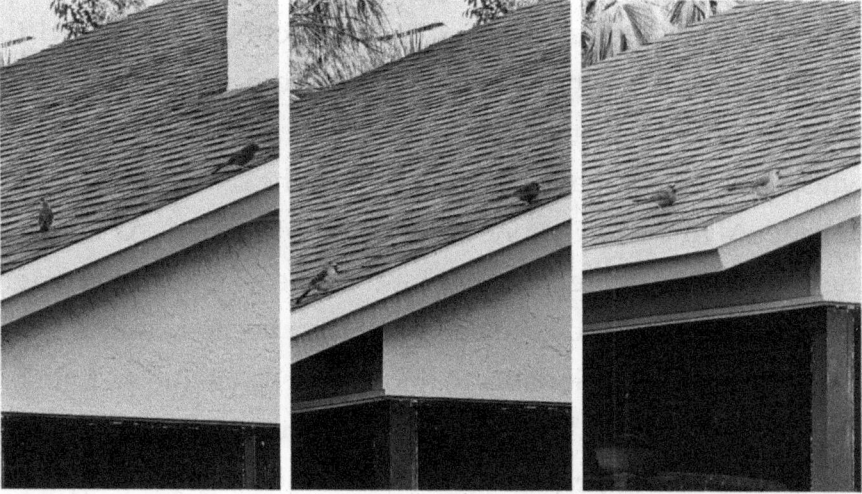

May 17, 2023

I have wind chimes on my lanai, and I rarely hear them. On this day, I was cleaning my house when I suddenly heard a faint chime. I paused and stepped toward the sliding glass doors, listening intently. Once again, one chime sounded. I opened the door to see if the wind was blowing but did not see any of the trees moving. Almost immediately, I felt a stir in my spirit and a whisper of energy that pulled me toward the screen door leading outside. All the while, more chimes began to sound. As I opened the screen door, there in front of me on the ground was a bright red cardinal, staring directly at me. It then began to dance in circles, stopping occasionally to look directly at me. At first, I thought it was Mom, until I learned that red cardinals are male. This had to be Clint, especially with the amount of dancing it was doing!

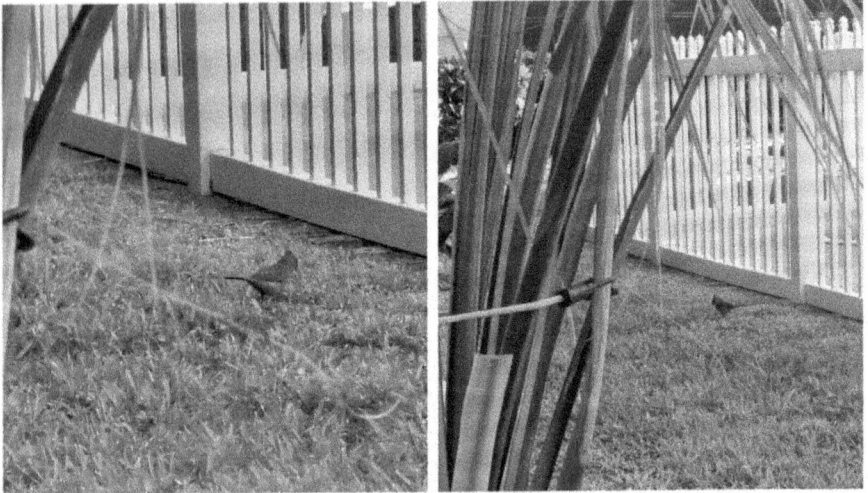

May 22, 2023

A few days later Renée reported that she saw a red cardinal perched on her fence in her front yard. She couldn't get to her phone in time to get a picture.

May 24, 2023

A few days after that, Karla reported that she also was visited by a beautiful red cardinal and shared this picture.

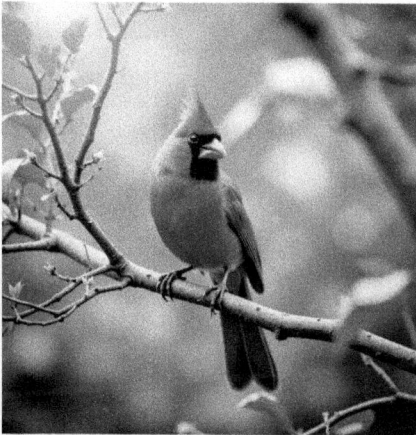

May 25, 2023

I would also like to share Kathy's post on Clint's legacy memorial website, which the funeral home established for friends and family to post. I had messaged Kathy to share with her our experiences we were having with seeing cardinals. I had not looked at the legacy board yet from the funeral. She then shared with me that she had posted a similar experience. Here is Kathy's post:

Legacy Reflection about Clint from Kathy

Dearest Clint,

On the day you went home to our lord, a cardinal visited me while I was walking in our neighborhood. For most of the walk, the cardinal flew a short distance ahead of me or to either side of me. I now believe that your heavenly spirit was embodied in the cardinal.

One of nature's most beautiful creations, cardinals symbolize love and devotion-the qualities that you abundantly shared with your family and friends during your time in the earthly realm.

While my heart overflows with sorrow for your loss, I rejoice that you now reside in Heaven, where you can once again dance, play the drums, and kick a soccer ball.

Thank you for sharing your "smart humor" with us during your time on Earth ("Glad you got to meet me"). Thank you for teaching us how to "stop and smell the roses" while enjoying the sunset. Thank you for loving my two sons Noah and Gabe as if they were your own. Thank you for being my forever friend.

In the midst of your suffering, you often exclaimed, "God is good-all the time," to which I added, "And all the time, God is good." You exemplified the principle of faith over fear. You frequently stated, "I know where I am going," alluding to Heaven after your time on Earth. Just as you were a guiding light in this world, I believe that you will become a guardian angel in the next.

With much love, Kathy"

She then shared another experience she had recently had:

Two nights ago, a cardinal perched in a tree across from Clint's old house. I stopped to admire the beautiful red bird, which looked intently at me and began warbling for about two minutes. I whispered, "I love you, Clint," and I think that he answered with additional singing. Soon after the cardinal flew right by me – at shoulder level – into the woods behind Clint's house. I am so glad that he is still watching over me."

March 17, 2024

I do believe when we die our energy remains present and our loved ones who have passed on visit us in various ways. I've recently had two dreams about Clint and one about Mom. Around February 2024 (10 months after they passed away), I dreamed that Mom and I were out driving around, and she was doing the driving. She was her young energetic self and, on a mission, to get through her checklist! She had no problem driving and dealing with the heavy traffic. Which was something she was no longer able to do after she had moved in with me in 2020. The mom in my dream—*that* was mom. This gave me confidence that she was no longer restrained in her earthly old body and she was back to her full energetic self.

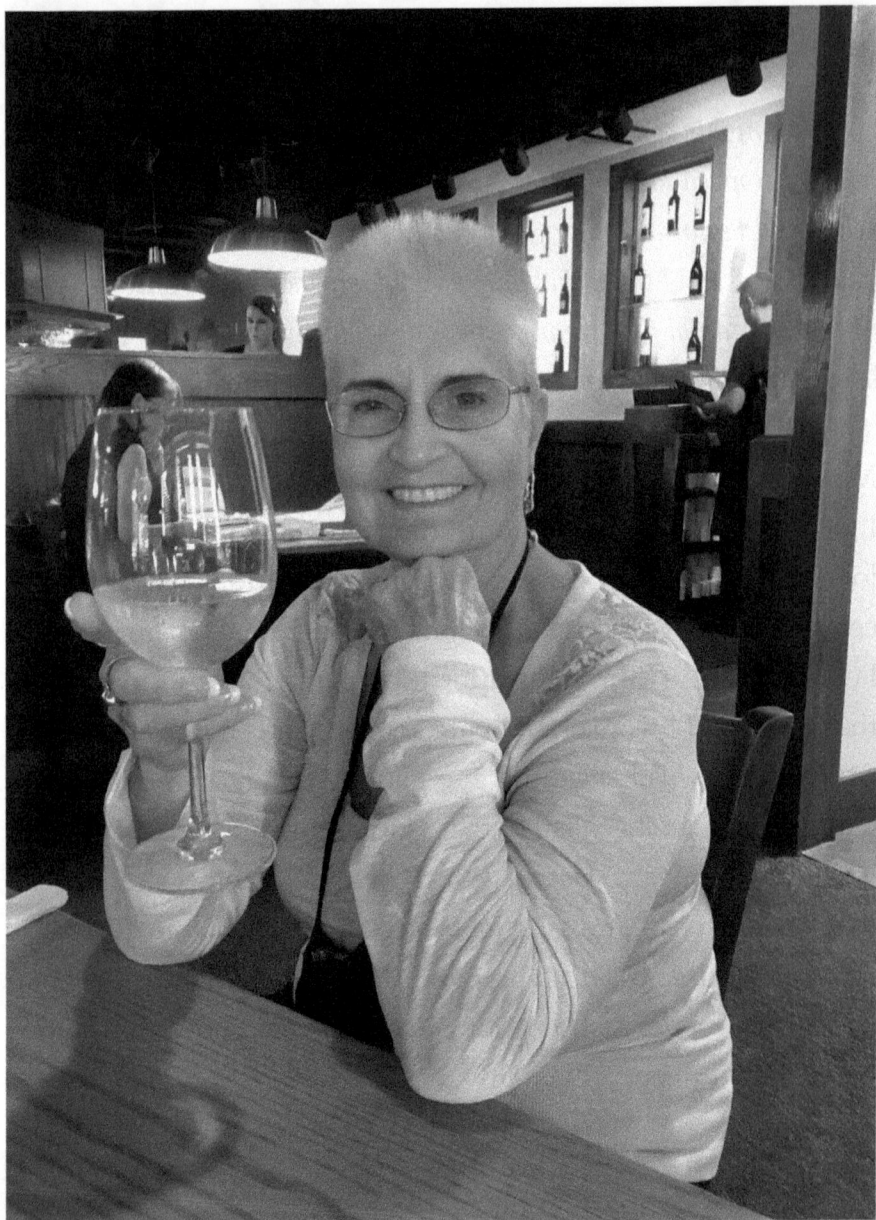

Mom toasting Karla

A few weeks later, I had a dream about Clint. In the dream, Renée and I were living in a run-down apartment building. I went for a walk. Whether it was the bad side of town, or the world had been through a disaster, the streets were crowded with homeless people. It was nighttime, and there were people hovering over barrel fires to keep warm. I passed by a group of individuals huddled around another homeless person casually lying on the ground and talking. He was dirty from head to toe, but I recognized the voice immediately: Clint! I yelled his name and tried to push through the people but couldn't. I ran back to the apartment to get Renée, who saw me through the window. I waved at her to come down. She couldn't get to me but instinctively knew to go to where Clint was. She found a spot in front of him, sat down, and started talking to him. I soon joined her and continued the conversation with Clint. It felt like he wasn't talking to us as his sisters but as though he was sharing wisdom about life. The dream ended there. I've tossed around what this dream could possibly mean. What I have settled on is that there is more to life and the afterlife as we know it. There is wisdom in all experiences, good or bad, and we must pay attention and learn from it.

On the morning of this journal entry (March 17, 2024, nearly 11 months after Clint passed away), I woke up remembering that night's dream. Charles and I had gone to bed in the dream, and as we dozed off, the bathroom light came on and we heard an electric razor. We both just "knew" it was Clint. We were excited, but we instinctively knew to just "wait"—to not get up and go see Clint. Soon after, Clint was standing beside my side of the bed. He pulled the covers up to my neck, tucking me in, smiling at me, then he leaned over and kissed my forehead. He then crawled into the bed next to me, rolled onto his side (away from me), pulled his covers up, and went to sleep. That, to me, was a very clear "Thank you!"

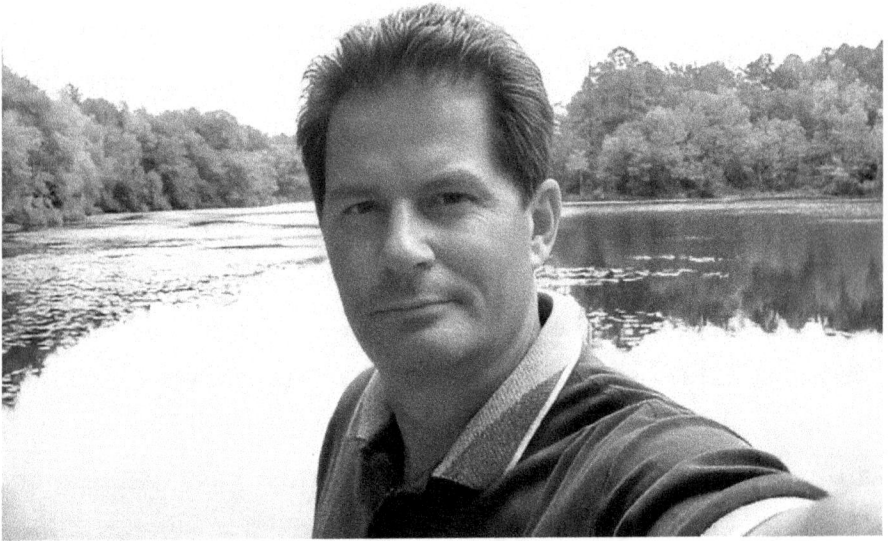

Clint by Daddy's Lake

After Your Loved Ones Are Gone

As I close out the final draft of this book, I see that we are approaching the two-year anniversary of Momma's and Clint's passing. I was able to close out both of their estates this year, with one last tax filing for Mom's that I still need to complete. Then my role as trustee will come to an end.

I still struggle with moments of anxiety as I find myself chasing a problem to solve. When I can't figure it out, I become frustrated with myself, and the negative self-talk ensues. But I continue to take another step forward. I continue to wake up and start my day, usually at the gym by 5 a.m. Exercise is good for the body, but even better for the mind. My siblings and I reach out to one another at least once a month, usually with Renée sending us a devotional for the day.

I do miss my lunch dates with Momma at Olive Garden. I also miss Daddy calling to tell me about how beautiful his garden is and then leaving me with some sappy dad jokes (his were hilarious country dad jokes!). I especially miss not getting to know my brother better and going dancing with him. I occasionally dream about each one, and sometimes when I'm driving around, I'll talk to them. I haven't heard a response yet, but I'm still listening.

ABOUT THE AUTHOR

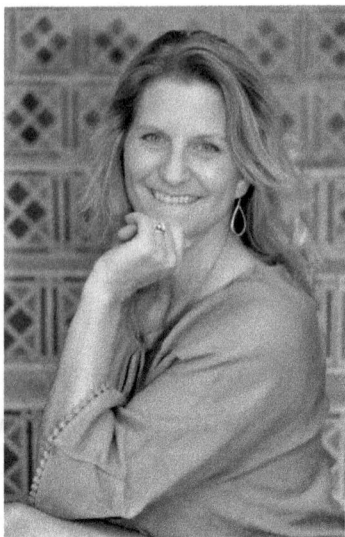

Julie Moore has spent much of her adult life serving her country in the U.S. Army. Born and raised in Jacksonville, Florida, Julie and her husband now reside in Southwest Florida. She has two children, Kate and Adam, and two grandchildren.

While serving in the military, Julie completed her master's degree in Performance Improvement and received a certification as a Black Belt in Lean Six Sigma. She retired with numerous meritorious awards, but her greatest reward was the many friendships she developed over the years.

Julie discovered journaling when she left home at the age of 18. Missing her family and friends she left behind she found comfort in writing about her daily routines, adventures, as well as new loves and losses. She continued this practice throughout her career and leaned on it heavily during her time as a caregiver. This book is the result of those writings of her experiences caring for her oldest brother and mother.

Although she would tell you that she doesn't have any hobbies, she does enjoy time with her family, the occasional quiet time alone, listening to nature like birds and waterfalls, a sip of fine bourbon, and dancing. She loves to dance!

www.ingramcontent.com/pod-product-compliance
Lightning Source LLC
Chambersburg PA
CBHW062126020426
42335CB00013B/1117